Reiki for Beginners

The Ultimate Guide to Reiki Healing, Tips for Reiki Meditation and Expand Mind Power, Increase Your Health and Positive Energy, Cleansing Aura and Self-Healing Techniques

Julia Crystal

This book is only a guide for beginners who want to learn and practice Reiki healing, meditation, and cleansing aura techniques as an alternative therapy. There are no health claims in using this book, such as curing certain health conditions.

Table of Content

Introduction _______________________________ *8*

Chapter 1 - Fundamentals of Reiki Healing_____ 10

What is Reiki Healing? ___________________ 10

Health Benefits of Reiki Healing ___________ 14

How to Balance Your Chakras with Reiki Healing__ 20

Applying Reiki to Your Daily Life ___________ 26

Chapter 2 - Reiki Meditation: How to Develop Positive Thinking ___________________ *31*

Expanding Your Mind Power _______________ 31

Ways to Increase Positive Thinking __________ 36

Restoring Balance to the Mind, Body, and Spirit ___ 41

Energy Flow Through the Meridian Lines of the Body ___________________________________ 47

Chapter 3 - Increase Your Health and Positive Energy ___________________________ *54*

How to Boost Your Immune System through Reiki _ 54

Best Daily Practices to Stay Happy and Healthy ___ 61

How to Practice Sleep-Focused Reiki__________ 65

Practicing Reiki to Relieve Stress _________________ 72

Chapter 4 - Cleansing Aura and Self-Healing Techniques _________________________________ 77

Reiki Healing Techniques to Master _____________ 77

How to Do Self-Healing at Home _______________ 83

Illnesses That Reiki Can Help With ____________ 88

How to Cleanse Your Aura ____________________ 94

Chapter 5 - Reiki and Nutrition ______________ 102

How to Use Reiki in Boosting Food Energy ______ 102

Why Ki Is Essential in the Food You Eat ________ 107

What to Do If You Forgot to Reiki Your Food _____112

The Power of Reiki Food Therapy _____________117

Chapter 6 - Interesting Facts About Reiki _____ 123

Who is Mikao Usui Sensei? ___________________ 123

What are the 5 Principles of Reiki? _____________ 128

Do Studies Approve of Reiki Healing? __________ 133

Is Reiki More Effective than Other Placebo Therapies? _________________________________ 138

Chapter 7 - Advanced Reiki Sessions: What to Expect ________________________________ 144

What is an Advanced Usui Reiki?________________ 144

How to Learn and Apply Advanced Reiki _________ 150

What Will You Experience During a Reiki Session? 153

From Whom Should You Receive Advanced Reiki? 160

Chapter 8 - Energy Medicine: The Future of Alternative Therapy ___________________________ **166**

What is Energy Medicine? _______________________ 166

Is Energy Medicine the Future of Health and Healing?
____ 171

Hospitals that Offer Energy Medicine____________ 177

Top Schools That Offer Energy Medicine Courses_ 182

Chapter 9 - Reiki Side Effects ___________________ **189**

Are There Side Effects of Reiki Healing__________ 189

Awkward Symptoms of Reiki Attunement _________ 195

Tips to Reduce the Side Effects of Reiki Attunements
____ 202

Tips to Protect Yourself When Doing Reiki _______ 207

Chapter 10 - How to Fix Leaking Energy and Close the Holes in Your Aura___________________ **213**

What is a Leaking Energy _______________________ 213

How to Fix Energy Leaks _______________________ 219

Tips to Maintain a Clean and Closed Aura _______ 224

Signs You Have Negative Entities Attached to You 229

Conclusion _______________________________ **236**

Introduction

Over the past one hundred years, Reiki has been the go-to healing therapy for spiritual people. They believe that each individual is guided by an invisible life force that controls physical, emotional, and mental well-being. Once the energy is flowing freely, you can harness your mind power and eliminate the obstructions such as stress overload, unhealed trauma, and negative thinking.

When you overcome those blockages, you can function again at a sub-optimal level. Nonbelievers may cringe at this, but people who consult Reiki masters often feel a positive aura after the healing therapy session. Generally, Reiki patients describe the sessions as grounding due to the calming effects of energy sweeping and light touch which controls the body's spiritual energy.

For you to achieve positive emotional realignment, Reiki practitioners undergo years of training to completely understand the healing power of subtle shifts of energy within the body. However, anyone can practice this alternative therapy by simply working with their own energy and impacting the flow of positive energy in other people.

Naturally, we want to stay healthy throughout our lifetime. Reiki can enhance your well-being and promote healing while enjoying deep relaxation through mind, body, and spirit. When you are healed and relaxed on the three levels, you can harmonize the chakras which can create a cleansing aura.

Chapter 1 - Fundamentals of Reiki Healing

What is Reiki Healing?

The term Reiki is derived from the Japanese words Rei (Higher Power or God's wisdom and Ki (life force energy). Reiki literally means spiritually guided life force energy.

Reiki healing is an alternative medicine that is more commonly known as energy healing. It uses a hands-on healing method called "palm healing" wherein the Reiki Master's universal energy is transferred to his patient for physical and emotional healing.

This Japanese healing technique is basically for relaxation and stress reduction. The main purpose is to promote healing without the use of modern medicines and medical procedures. From the palm of the healer, a life force energy is passed onto the patient, giving positive energy to cure negative thoughts and other stressful elements.

If your life force energy decreases, then you're more likely to feel stress and get sick. On the other hand, if you keep this energy at a high level, you can stay healthy and happy. Reiki can treat you wholly, including your body, soul, mind, and emotions. By increasing and allowing your life force energy to flow through you, the beneficial effects are relaxation, security, peaceful mind, and well-being.

Unlike other medical treatments, Reiki is a natural and safer technique for self-healing and spiritual improvement you can use in the long run. For over a hundred years, this simple healing method has been effective in providing beneficial effects for common illnesses such as pain and anxiety.

Moreover, this healing technique also helps boost the effectiveness of medical procedures to reduce the side effects and relieve the symptoms. Reiki has been helpful in promoting fast recoveries in patients with various ailments. Some doctors are now recognizing the importance of this natural alternative to medical techniques.

You can learn this technique by attending a Reiki class or training. This healing power is transferred through a process called attunement wherein the life force energy is passed from the palm of the practitioner to the student for you to enhance one's quality of life as well as overall health.

However, the use of this ability is not limited to the spiritual development or intellectual capacity of an individual. Rather, it's available to anyone who wants to practice spiritually guided life force energy. Through so many decades, it's been successfully practiced by people of any age and background.

Reiki may be spiritual, but it's not a religious belief or anything of that kind. In fact, it doesn't follow church doctrine nor ask you to believe in something to learn how to use Reiki. This healing technique doesn't depend on any beliefs, it works regardless of your religion. Since Reiki comes from the Higher wisdom of God, you may find that receiving life force energy brings you closer to your religion instead of the intellectual idea of it.

Despite Reiki not being a religion, it's still essential to act and live in such a manner that helps harmonize your relationship with other people. In practicing this natural healing method, you need some ethical ideals for you to improve harmony and peace.

Adding your ideals to Reiki healing can develop better spiritual balance when tapping into your life force energy. During the experience, the main goal is to make you realize that spiritual healing through conscious self-improvement is essential in the success of receiving Reiki.

Lasting healing energies can be achieved by accepting that you are responsible for healing. Therefore, you should be actively taking part in the entire experience as you receive the Reiki energy. With active commitment and willingness to improve yourself, it's easier to complete the process and get positive results. Remember, the ideals will serve as guidelines in living a graceful life while the virtues are essential in understanding your inherent value.

Health Benefits of Reiki Healing

As an ancient healing technique, Reiki has been proven to produce impressive results through energy transfer, positive mindsets, and gentle touch. Whether you're receiving Reiki for spirituality development, energy balance, or trauma healing, this method offers endless benefits.

Here are some of the most common Reiki healing benefits that you can get:

- Harmony and balance. The non-invasive method of transferring energy helps promote overall health and well-being. The body restores the balance throughout the body, mind, and soul which creates harmony to support people in living an optimistic lifestyle.

- Pressure relief. If you need to release some tension in your muscles, Reiki healing will allow you to relax and relieve all these pressures from your body. In as fast as two minutes, you can get pure relaxation by clearing your mind and relieving stress. Reiki's energy transfer helps people feel lighter and more peaceful to make it possible to connect with the inner self and reflect on life.

- Overcome energy blocks. With regular Reiki healing, you can consistently keep your energy flow clear from all negativity. Unlocking the flow of life force energy in your body allows you to enhance memory and learning, reduce physical pain, promote mental sharpness, and feel less stressed. Maintaining the energy passageways unblocked also gives you positive energy which prevents mood swings, pain, anger, and fear.

- Stronger immune system. The techniques used in Reiki healing cleanses the body from toxins by assisting in its self-healing state. Once this state is stimulated, your body will begin to rid of all the useless energies. This allows you to develop a strong immune system that is protected from burnout and exhaustion.

- Improved focus. Reiki helps you to simply be in the current time. You receive positive energy to focus your mind on the present rather than the past. With an improved focus, you can reduce the worries and anxieties about what's going to happen in the future. By being in the present moment, you learn to accept your life as it unfolds. As a result, you create a positive response to circumstances and people.

- Better sleep. The best thing about Reiki healing is that you are guaranteed to feel relaxed after each session. It helps your body to develop a healthy sleep pattern. In return, the body can heal better while the mind can think more clearly. If the mind is at ease after a Reiki healing therapy, you can sleep better.

- Spiritual growth. Emotional cleansing is essential in developing spiritual growth. Reiki healing addresses the body, mind, and spirit for you to ensure the person heals both the physical and spiritual being. Meaning, the life force energy that is transferred through a Reiki session helps in boosting the mood and attitude of the receiver towards living a better life.

- Self-healing ability. To go back to a near-natural state, the internal body systems are balanced through Reiki healing. This improves bodily systems including your blood pressure, heart rate, breathing, and circulation. With a normal balance within the body, it allows you to develop self-healing ability.

- Reduced anxiety. More research is needed to prove the effectiveness of Reiki healing, but this natural therapy can reduce anxieties as well as fatigue. According to a study conducted in 2015, people undergoing cancer treatment were also given distant Reiki to help improve medical care. The results include lowered pain levels, fatigue, and anxiety.

- Relieve depression. Reiki healing can also be used in managing depressive episodes. In fact, there are depression treatment plans that include this energy healing method. A study conducted in 2010 showed that Reiki can improve physical symptoms in adults with depression. The participants have seen improvements in their mood and wellness. In addition, they were able to relax more, enhance self-care, and increase curiosity.

These benefits of Reiki healing can help people enhance their overall well-being. With better self-confidence, sleep patterns, and mood, you will notice that you become more relaxed and calm. The inner peace you can get from Reiki therapy may be enough to improve your quality of life.

If you have certain health conditions such as tension, headache, insomnia, and nausea, Reiki can reduce these symptoms. The feeling of relaxation you experience during a Reiki session can benefit your health. Not to mention, this non-invasive healing method is generally safe so there's nothing to worry about any harmful side effects. However, Reiki should never be used as a substitute for any treatment plan recommended by your health professional.

There are plenty of ways to benefit from Reiki healing. It doesn't just target one problem in your body, but it helps treat everything at the same time. As a powerful healing tool, energy transfer can cure all elements and symptoms of one particular condition. However, it's important to work with a certified Reiki master to get all these benefits.

If you have blocked chakras, Reiki healing can help you balance your inner energies and alleviate the symptoms. By channeling life force energy from the palm of the Reiki master to the receiver's, it's easy to identify the blockages and open them to allow the positive energy to flow throughout the body.

Physical pain from an injury can be reduced by targeting Reiki to the seven chakras, the body's central energy that aligns the spine. However, this is not overnight healing. The pains and imbalances in the body will take some time to be balanced with the chakras for you to experience relief.

The following are the major problems linked to your chakras that can be treated by a Reiki practitioner:

- Root Chakra. The root chakra is found at the lowest part of your spine. It is linked to problems including survival, identity, and Earth connection. An imbalanced root chakra can be related to financial security and personal fears. Some physical symptoms include chronic pain on the lower back, ankles, feet, calves, knees, legs, hips, and the groin. With Reiki healing targeted at your root chakra, it gives a sense of feeling supported and grounded.

- Crown Chakra. This chakra is found at the central part of your head, hence the name. The crown chakra is your connection to your spirituality, divine guidance, and the universe. By performing Reiki to open this chakra, you can develop a sense of safety, oneness, and trust in the universe.

- Third-eye chakra. The third-eye chakra is found between your eyebrows. It gives you extrasensory to see what the naked eye can't. Basically, your intuition lies in this chakra including your psychic perception and clairvoyance. An imbalanced third-eye chakra can cause difficulty in trusting your insights.

Reiki healing can cleanse this chakra for you to help you control your inner knowing.

- Throat chakra. Known to help people speak their truth, the throat chakra is found at the lower part of your throat. Imbalances in this chakra may cause sore throat and thyroid issues. If you have obstructed throat chakra, emotional manifestations may include fear of being rejected and judged. To unblock your throat chakra, Reiki can be performed to help you express yourself freely and voice out your truth.

- Heart chakra. This chakra is found at the central part of your chest. It helps you speak your mind and express how you actually feel. An imbalanced heart chakra can make you resentful, disconnected from yourself and other people, and feel lonely. Reiki healing can make you more open to love and be compassionate to others.

- Solar plexus chakra. This chakra is your power center that connects to your self-protection and self-esteem. Solar plexus chakra is found two inches above your navel. Some common signs that this chakra is blocked include whirling sensation, discomfort, and low energy. Physically, you will feel bloated, constipated, or exhausted. To treat these symptoms, Reiki can remove the blockages in your navel area to promote self-healing and overall wellness.

- Sacral chakra. As the opposite of the solar plexus chakra, this chakra is found two inches below your navel. This is linked to creativity, procreation, gender, and sex. An imbalanced sacral chakra can be manifested by painful hip, pelvic, or lower back. Some common causes of blockages in this chakra include trauma and sexual abuse. Reiki can release these traumas to help you heal and begin life anew.

Aside from Reiki healing techniques, you can also eat chakra-balancing foods to improve your chakras. Other ways to maintain balanced energy within your body is to use essential oils and practice chakra meditation on a regular basis. You can also perform Kundalini yoga to clear all those blockages in your chakras.

If you are interested in adding chakra-balancing foods to your diet, here are some tips you can follow:

- For root chakra, you can add root vegetables such as carrots, potatoes, radishes, turnips, ginger, onions, garlic, and celery to your meals. Red plants are also helpful such as beets, cranberries, pomegranate, tomatoes, strawberries, raspberries, and red peppers.

- For sacral chakra, you can add yellow and orange foods such as sweet potatoes, oranges, and carrots to your diet. Other essential foods for sacral chakra include coconuts, seeds, nuts, and fish.

- For solar plexus chakra, you can add yellow foods such as pineapples, lemons, banana, corn, yellow peppers, and garbanzo beans. Other healthy foods for your solar plexus chakra include rice, oats, and other whole grains.

- For heart chakra, you can add green foods such as chlorophyll, asparagus, celery, avocado, spinach, kiwi, and kale to your daily meals.

- For throat chakra, you can add blueberries, blackberries, echinacea, ginseng, apricots, and pears to your meals.

- For third-eye chakra, you can add chia seeds, red grapes, purple cabbage, eggplant, and plums to your daily nutrition.

- For crown chakra, you can add white foods such as onion, garlic, mushrooms, chamomile, and coconut to your diet. Don't forget to drink plenty of water to keep your crown chakra well balanced.

Healthy chakras mean they are not underactive nor overactive. A simple change in your diet can help improve and balance your chakras. This is important in boosting the positive energy as well as the health benefits you can get from Reiki healing.

Applying Reiki to Your Daily Life

Every day, it's important to feel each blessing and be grateful even for the simple things you have. You need to have a positive outlook in life to do the things that are meaningful to you. The spiritual healing art of Reiki will help you channel positive energy to allow yourself to heal from physical, emotional, and spiritual difficulties.

Applying Reiki to daily life is so simple because life force energy flows through every living thing. You can connect with anyone using your healing energy while strengthening the energy in others. Helping other people is a great way to create harmony among living things.

To jump-start your day, set your alarm clock at least 10 minutes in advance so you can hit snooze just once. If you hit snooze several times, you will miss this essential first step to Reiki application in daily life. Once you've hit snooze, put your palm on any part of your body to begin channeling Reiki. For 10 minutes, you can feel the positive energy flowing through your body.

You can activate your Reiki symbols if you have any. Put them in your hand by drawing the symbols on it. Some even draw their symbols on their mouth using their tongue. But if you want to keep it simple, you can just visualize the symbols on your mind. You don't need to perform all those hand positions since you only have very limited time.

You can put your hand on any body part to start self-healing. During the energy transfer, relax and focus on the life force energy that is flowing from your hand to the area where it's needed. Enjoy the remaining 9 minutes as your alarm clock goes off. After this, you will surely feel good about yourself and begin your day with a smile on your face.

If your mind is working nonstop and you want to quiet your thoughts, put your hands together and hold them in front of your chest. This is called the Gasho position wherein you focus on your middle fingers as they meet. While doing that, you recognize any thoughts that you have and then dismiss them to concentrate again on your middle fingers. Doing Gasho meditation on a regular basis can help you relax and re-balance your life.

Another Reiki activity you can do daily is energizing your room. This is more helpful in charging meeting rooms so everyone can feel positive energy and become more productive and optimistic while performing today's tasks. State your intentions and hold your hands upwards to allow the energy to flow out. You can do this without them knowing by simply bringing a cup and holding it up when you drink so the Reiki energy is sent to the conference room.

However, if you have symbols, you can draw or visualize them for you to energize the room. Use mental symbols to help keep emotions and interactions under control throughout the meeting. If you think your next meeting would be difficult, you can do Reiki in the room so that it will turn alright once it's adjourned.

Do you watch television every day? It's another perfect opportunity to energize your body. Put your hand on any part of the body to do Reiki. You can also activate your symbols if you have them. Again, you don't need to perform all those hand positions because you only have a few minutes to do Reiki while watching TV.

Rather, you can hold your hands on a specific part of the body where Reiki is needed. This will help you stay relaxed while waiting for the commercials to finish, so you can watch your favorite show again. Soaking yourself up on the Reiki energy will divert your attention from being bothered by long TV ads to staying laid-back on your couch throughout the show.

Now, if you're taking medications or supplements, you can energize them to help the pills become more effective. Giving your medications Reiki energy will support the body in accepting the medicines with much better potency. You can also activate your symbols while energizing your supplements and vitamins. This is more helpful if you are currently dealing with emotional issues while taking your medication.

Hold the bottle of pills and state your intentions while allowing the energy to flow through it. You may ask for divine guidance that your medicines be effective in treating your medical condition. In addition, concerns about any potential side effects will be lessened by simply doing a Reiki on the bottles before taking your vitamins. You can do this every time you take your pills to see significant improvement in your overall health.

Chapter 2 - Reiki Meditation: How to Develop Positive Thinking

Expanding Your Mind Power

The value and strength of Reiki healing can be developed more by simply observing a few guidelines. Since the energy comes from a bottomless source, Reiki contains overflowing spiritual power and loving wisdom. There's no limit when it comes to the benefits you can get from this energy healing technique. Therefore, it's possible to expand your mind power by following these guidelines.

First of all, you need to believe that it works and it's right for you. Knowing in your heart that Reiki is an effective healing technique for your entire being can help improve the results you're seeking. Also, it's important to consider the flow of energy you're receiving within a specific environment. The quality of the room can affect Reiki healing treatments as well as the results. Make sure your room has ideal temperature, not too cold nor too hot.

The windows in the room should be open to allow some fresh air inside and provide better ventilation. It should not be stuffy or filled with unnecessary things that can attract negative psychic energy. Before the treatment, burn some sage to expel any negative energy inside the room. While the smoke is diffusing in the room, you can call in your Reiki guides, ascended masters, and ancestors to bless and help you during the healing treatment.

Some even put images of Dr. Hayashi and Dr. Usui in the room to feel their presence and guidance. If you have essential oils, flowers, or incense, they can also help increase the vibration in the room. Moving into a receptive mental state can be more effective with some soothing music, too.

Before the treatment, the Reiki master should sit in a meditating position with hands on the legs while doing Reiki. After several minutes, the dominant hand is used to draw the power symbol of Reiki on the floor, ceiling, and each wall of the room.

During the energy transfer, it's helpful to recite something like you're blessing the room with energy and light. Recite it three times on the wall, ceiling, and floor to strengthen the Reiki energy. Draw another Reiki power symbol in the central part of your room. This will send energy into your room so it will be filled with the needed healing energy.

Here's a more elaborate way to start expanding your mind through Reiki meditation:

- Before the treatment, the palm chakras should be energized by putting or drawing the master and power symbols on the hand. This will open your chakras on your hands while transferring Reiki energy.

- Draw another power symbol on your belly area, but this time the symbol should be a little bigger to empower and protect you. Then put smaller Reiki power symbols on every chakra in your body to complete the healing.

- Put each symbol into your crown chakra so it passes through your heart before raising the vibration. This will make the Reiki symbols' energy more accessible and effective.

One interesting fact about Reiki healing is that the energy continues to flow no matter what you're thinking or doing in your mind. You can even talk to someone about anything, such as trivial matters and gossips while on your phone. The source and receiver of the energy will still get the benefits they need to heal and relax their mind, body, and spirit.

However, divided attention may not give you the best result. Remember that your focus on the spiritual experience is essential in giving Reiki the most effective healing. Therefore, you need to give Reiki the reverence for you to get the most benefits from this energy healing technique.

f you meditate instead of talking while allowing the energy to flow through you, you will experience increased life force energy more instantly. During Reiki meditation, the energy merges with the mind therefore leading to a more harmonized energy flow. As a result, Reiki flows more freely throughout your body where it's particularly needed.

Also while meditating, there will be some currents of energy felt in different parts of the body such as the hands, arms, spine, and chakras. Some people even feel vibrations, heat, pulsations, and other soothing sensations as the energy flows through them. You can use your inner eye to see the energy flowing through you. The Reiki energy may look like particles of golden, white, or other colors of light passing through each chakra.

As you experience this state of mind along with the vibrations, your mind becomes more optimistic. As you feel uplifted, it expands your mind power while channeling peace, spiritual love, and joy. You may also perceive positive visions and fantasies as your mind elevates to a higher spiritual plane. Go inward and look up to your Crown chakra for you to mentally travel to the main source of the energy and unify with it.

Ways to Increase Positive Thinking

Positive thinking is your mental attitude towards beneficial thoughts, images, and words that promote success and self-growth. A positive mind cultivates health, joy, and contentment in life. It anticipates successful outcomes from every action and situation. What the mind looks for, it finds. However, you need to make an effort to succeed in whatever you want in life.

Reiki meditation gives you experiences that are deeply healing and gratifying at the same time. It also helps open the pathways wherein Reiki energy flows for you to increase positive thinking. So what are the best ways to gain more sensational thoughts while you meditate and receive Reiki energy?

Adding some prayers during the Reiki treatment can effectively increase the strength and flow of energy. Praying can be done mentally or out loud for you to boost positive thinking. You can call on your ascended masters, spirit guides, angels, Krishna, Buddha, or Jesus to ask for direction and healing. While praying, ask the Supreme Being to strengthen your Reiki and bless you with a happy and healthy life.

Accept that there's no boundary to the healing power and value that's accessible to you. With your prayers, use these techniques to effectively merge with the Reiki energy and feel it while it passes through your body. By simply adding prayers to your treatment, it makes you feel more powerful and helps gain positive thoughts that can lead to better visions for ultimate happiness and wellness.

Some of the exercises you can do to help develop your Ki and open the pathways for the energy to flow freely are Tai Chi and Chi Gong. The pathways they open are actually the same where the Reiki energy flows. According to Reiki masters, practicing these moving meditation exercises can help strengthen your Reiki. In fact, those who practice Tai Chi have a stronger life force energy than people who don't.

Regular Tai Chi or Chi Gong is generally healthy and can also improve your Reiki. In addition, you can use affirmations and self-hypnosis to increase positive thinking. Make suggestions to yourself to support stronger healing results and believe that it's working on your body, mind, and soul. With positive thinking, you can get what you want and it will be for your overall well-being.

When you apply the "mind over matter" saying to your life, then there's nothing impossible for you. There is no limitation to what you can do and achieve if you have a positive mind. It's also important to keep in mind that Reiki healing has its own consciousness. When you intentionally improve the energy and value you allow to flow through you, it creates a mind that is boundless. There's absolute power in someone who thinks he can do anything.

The following are some effective ways to increase positive thinking:

- Recognize any negative thoughts and take action to forget them before they settle down in your brain. If your mood is going low, do things that can uplift you such as listening to good music, hugging your family, playing with your pets, or taking a walk with nature. Do anything that diverts your attention from negativity.

- Spend more time with your friends and family who uplift your mood. Positive thinking is contagious, the more you hang out with positive people the better you can manage a positive mindset.

- Watch out for your own habits. Are you exercising regularly, eating healthy food, and drinking plenty of water? These simple things are essential in creating a positive attitude.

- De-clutter and organize your things at home. Surrounding yourself with essential things and letting go of those that dull your light is important. What you keep in your space should make you feel happy including books, artworks, houseplants, framed photos, and even healing crystals.

- If someone says you won't succeed at anything, take it as a challenge. Work hard so you can prove them wrong. Sometimes, people are telling you things that they themselves are afraid to do. When you succeed, make it an inspiration for others to be successful.

- Volunteer for charities and communities with like-minded individuals. There's nothing more motivating than doing things with people who have common goals. Helping others also gives you a spiritual and emotional high that can help you lead a positive life.

- Take time to de-stress no matter how busy you are. If you are always stressed out, it will eventually take its toll on you. As early as now, make sure to recharge yourself by enjoying a time alone or getting a massage. However, the best thing to relieve stress is to perform some Reiki meditation.

It's easy to start on these activities, but doing it consistently is the real challenge. So, how far are you willing to go to develop and maintain a positive mind?

Restoring Balance to the Mind, Body, and Spirit

Perhaps the first thing that comes to your mind when you think about wellness is healthy food. While this is true, exercise and diet are not the only requirements for being healthy. You also need to nurture your mind and spirit for you to maintain your health.

The body and mind are interconnected, which means they have an effect on each other. For instance, if you're stressed, it can give you headaches and other forms of physical pain. Chronic stress can even lead to serious illnesses. Therefore, you need to be mindful of what you allow in your mind so that your body will not suffer the consequences.

Restoring balance to your mind, body, and spirit is essential in nurturing yourself physically, mentally, emotionally, and spiritually. There are a lot of things to help you attain overall wellness. Below are only some of the best ways to cultivate mind-body-spirit balance:

- Make it a habit to read everyday. Learning is an unending process because life doesn't stop teaching us. Besides, the world continues to evolve and you need to keep up with those changes. Once you graduate, you will realize that the real world has more lessons to teach you than in your classroom. Reading, attending workshops, watching documentaries, and taking an online class are excellent ways to learn.

- Meditate regularly. Reiki meditation helps improve your mood, sleep, memory, and creativity. You only need a few minutes to meditate and you will experience its benefits immediately.

- Avoid living a sedentary lifestyle. Sitting all day is bad for your health as it can lead to a shortened lifespan, diabetes, and heart disease. Standing and moving around even during a busy day at work is important in your overall well-being.

- Exercise regularly. Spend 15 minutes everyday to exercise, from moderate to fast workout. If your workplace is walking distance from home, you can ride a bike or simply walk on specific days. Exercising is essential for physical stamina, mood, and heart health.

- Make time to see nature. Spending time outside is an instant mood booster. You can hike, camp, play outdoor sports, or attend a gathering in your community with friends and colleagues. The feeling of being close to nature is a healthy way to keep grounded.

- Eat a plant-based diet. Are you eating lots of greens lately? How does it affect your body? Fruits and vegetables can keep you safe from chronic diseases including cancer. When buying food, you can shop from the farmer's market to find in-season produce at a good price. Plus, the wet market offers fresh products that are healthy for you.

- Join an activism group. If you're involved in volunteer organizations, you will realize how the world needs people like you. Using your voice to seek justice for others and help the poor get support from the government is truly life-changing. Remember, we are all connected. And in that connectedness, we can achieve our common goals.

- Pursue your passions. Aside from working and being successful in your career, you also need to find time to do what keeps you passionate. Fueling your passions helps make your spirit happy. When the spirit is happy, your mind and body are also happy. Some things to keep you passionate include painting, dancing, making music, writing, gardening, and swimming.

- Be grateful and kind. Make a list of the things that you are grateful for such as food, good health, shelter, friends, and family. This will remind you how beautiful life is. Also, be kind to others and yourself. Treat people the way you want to be treated. It's important in maintaining a healthy balance to your mind, body, and spirit because a grateful and kind soul has a huge physical and mental impact on your overall well-being.

- Get more sleep and pamper yourself. Every night, you should get at least 8 hours of sleep to recharge your body for the next day. When doing your skincare routine, make sure to choose natural beauty products to avoid harsh chemicals that are absorbed by the body.

- Build a career that you've always dreamed of. Your career path should not just be about earning money, it should also help you pursue your dreams. A meaningful career will surely last longer than a job that only gives you temporary happiness.

There are so many things you can do to restore balance to your mind, body, and soul. No matter what you want to do, always keep a good heart so that your mind and body will follow through. Reiki treatment can help maintain balance in your entire being so that you can pursue your goals and succeed.

Life force energy nourishes and sustains your body while supporting and increasing your self-healing ability. This is important in speeding up recovery from injuries and illnesses. If there's a balance between your mind, body, and spirit, you can heal not just physically, but also emotionally and psychologically.

Energy Flow Through the Meridian Lines of the Body

The meridian lines of the body refer to the energy network consisting of lines or channels wherein the life force energy flows. Your life energy or Ki is transported through these channels, but it's not a physical structure such as the circulatory system. Rather, it's a process in which Reiki practitioners study just like how western doctors study the human anatomy.

Common blockages in the meridian lines include bad diet, trauma, injury, alcohol or drug abuse, and stress. These are all related to the main causes of health problems today. The flow of energy through these lines helps condition your overall existence such as how you feel, how you think, and how your body moves.

Life - force energy is distributed to the 12 regular meridian lines of the body in these rhythms:

- From your chest area, which then passes through the lungs, heart, pericardium to your hands.

- From your arms, which then passes through the large intestines and small intestines to your head.

- From your head, which then passes through the gall bladder, stomach, and bladder to your feet.

- From your feet, which then passes through the kidney, liver, and spleen back to your chest area for you to complete the cycle.

If there's a problem in a specific organ or channel, it can be treated by following the energy flow and rhythm. From that specific part of the body, you can do Reiki healing to cure an injury or health issue. However, aside from the primary channels, there are these so-called extraordinary meridians that you also need to learn.

Each extraordinary meridian has a specific function which further helps understand the links between them. They serve as energy and blood reservoirs that are regulated whenever the primary channels need them. Below are the main functions of the extraordinary meridians:

- Distribute the "essence" throughout the body since the extraordinary meridians are strongly connected to your kidneys.

- Circulate the protective Ki through the torso for you to maintain good health.

- Since the body's meridian system is an intricate network of interconnected energy lines, mastering it can help you understand the energy flow of Ki through your body.

If you want to maintain harmony and balance in your meridians, it's important that your body is at peace.

An imbalance can disrupt your health, therefore causing certain illnesses to manifest. To use Reiki treatment for healing such body problems require accessing these energy points. It will help release all the blockages that are causing the imbalance.

Reiki therapy can also help restore your body's natural equilibrium which is essential in aiding good health. The hands-on approach of this energy healing technique balances physical health and emotional well-being. This natural treatment releases repressed emotional traumas for you to relieve the body from bodily symptoms including chronic pain and headaches.

Generally, taking care of your bladder meridian is the ultimate way to maintain balance in your life. The bladder is actually the longest meridian in the body, touching every organ and system. Meaning, you need to work on this meridian for you to distribute balanced energies throughout other meridian lines. A harmonious and balanced bladder meridian is equal to a healthy mind, body, and spirit.

Working along with the bladder is the kidney. They are responsible for keeping a healthy supply of fluid in your body while expelling toxins that cause chronic diseases. The bladder significantly affects your autonomic nervous system, waste elimination, perspiration, sexual fluids, lymphatic flow, cell lubrication, and blood circulation.

The bladder holds chronic stress and tension as this meridian runs through your back, hence storing negative energies in it. You can open up your bladder meridian by maintaining flexibility in the spine so that the energy can release all the tensions and stress. It can show you specific areas in your life where you are negative and not flexible. Determining these areas will help you move forward with wisdom and courage.

Symbolically, the bladder meridian represents your past and your unconscious self as well as the aspects in yourself that you can't see. The meridian channels of the bladder pass through your pelvic area, including the ovaries, testicles, uterus, and prostate;

therefore, it affects your sexuality. The life force energy develops in your bladder and is stored in your kidneys.

Below are helpful tips to nourish your bladder and keep it healthy:

- Drink more water daily.

- Avoid too much sugar, caffeinated drinks, drugs, chocolate, and salty foods.

- Keep your body flexible through regular exercises.

- Get at least 8 hours of sleep every night.

- Breathe deeply and stretch your spinal column.

- Consume more stir-fry, sauté, and steamed veggies.

- Drink warm beverages in the morning.

- Eat healthy foods such as walnuts, green beans, onions, lettuce, carrots, water chestnuts, raspberries, chives, eggplants, celery, watermelon, strawberries, pears, and grapes.

While working on your meridian lines and physical flexibility, it's also important to gain emotional and mental flexibility to balance your mind, body, and soul.

Chapter 3 - Increase Your Health and Positive Energy

How to Boost Your Immune System through Reiki

Seasonal ailments including flu and colds are common during cold months. While the immune system is fending off the doubling presence of viruses and bacteria, it can weaken at the same time. The good news is that you can help your body heal from these illnesses by undergoing Reiki sessions.

The following are the main health benefits of Reiki non-invasive healing:

- Increase physical and healing energy.

- Enhance immune function.

- Promote spiritual growth.

- Boost relaxation.

- Reduce stress.

Reiki is an effective healing technique that works physically, mentally, emotionally, and spiritually. With more studies conducted on the effectiveness of Reiki healing, it's starting to be recognized as a great alternative for medical treatments across the globe.

Stress is the main reason why your life force energy or Ki gets disrupted. It weakens your body's ability to fight off viruses, bacteria, and other threats. Therefore, you are more likely to develop diseases including the number one cause of death in America – heart disease. Other common problems you might develop from a weakened immune system are diabetes, skin issues, respiratory problems, and digestive disorders.

According to the American Institute of Stress, approximately 75 to 95 percent of hospital visits are due to chronic stress. On average, 80 percent of health concerns including pain and illnesses are due to stress. The hormones released in your body when you're stressed also affect sleep and can potentially damage specific areas of the brain that are linked to memory. Some of the most common causes of stress include distrust, anger, fear, and worry.

With Reiki sessions, you can unblock the self-healing ability of your body so that it can restore and regenerate the immune system. A strong immunity helps increase your white blood cells (WBCs) that prevent diseases and infections. To strengthen your immune system, you need to avoid stress, exercise regularly, and eat nutritious foods.

Experiencing deep relaxation through Reiki can reduce stress and release tensions in the body. It can help you manage your stressors and boost your self-healing ability without expensive medications. Doing Reiki regularly is an excellent preventative measure as it helps keep your immune system in a more stable condition.

Energy healing stabilizes WBC count and increases it when needed. The WBCs immediately act when there's an infection entering the body. They surround the area where viruses and bacteria are present for you to produce antibodies that will kill all these microorganisms. While WBCs are always on alert mode, they may get defeated by the viruses once they are low in number. This is why it's important to keep stress at bay so that your immune system stays strong and the WBCs remain at high levels.

Now, is there a scientific explanation of the effectiveness of Reiki healing on your immune system?

There are many studies conducted by expert researchers to find out the effects of doing Reiki on people's immunity. The first-ever study on Reiki had 45 healthy respondents that were grouped into three, with 15 members each: No Treatment group, Reiki Treatment group, and Placebo Treatment group which was assisted by an individual who just imitated what the Reiki master did because he didn't know anything about Reiki.

The researchers measured the effects by using their own tools that allowed them to determine how the nervous system functioned during the treatment. They measured and recorded the heartbeat, breathing activity, stress, arousal, emotion's psychological index, and cardiac vagal sound.

To compare the results, the researchers considered the before and after values of each group. The conclusion stated that the heart rate and diastolic blood pressure significantly decreased in the Treatment group, the respondents who actually received Reiki from a knowledgeable master. Between the Placebo group and No Treatment group, significant quantitative differences were recorded.

The most interesting part about these studies on Reiki's effects is that practitioners are able to release biological improvements in their treatments instead of just creating a feeling of wellness.

Your immune system needs to be balanced and harmonized for you to function well. The life force energy or Ki should flow throughout your physical body to avoid blocked chakras or meridian channels. You are likely to get sick when there's an imbalance in your energy flow. A free-flowing Ki will help you maintain good health and overall well-being through regular Reiki sessions.

Here are some breathing techniques to enhance your immune function:

- Activate your life force energy and focus symbol.

- Put your hand on your thymus while the other is placed on your upper navel area.

- Focus on your thymus chakra.

- Imagine, activate, or draw the focus symbol in your front with the length of your arm.

- Imagine, activate, or draw the focus symbol at the center of your body's chakra.

- Imagine, activate, or draw the focus symbol on your back with the length of your arm.

- Breathe in to send light from the focus symbol on your front while allowing your breath to pass through your body until it reaches the focus symbol on your back.

- Breathe out to send light from your back to your front chakra. Do this several times and then inhale and exhale normally.

This is a powerful practice to integrate the energy channels for you to release blockages that are weakening your immune system. You can do this regularly, especially during times when you can get a good rest afterward.

The deep state of relaxation you experience through a Reiki session is essential in removing energy blockages, reducing stress, restoring and boosting your overall wellness. If you want to create long-term positive change in your life, practicing Reiki every day is the first step.

Starting your day with a motivating daily practice is key to a happy and healthy life. So, how do you usually begin your day?

Daily practice refers to the routine you religiously do every single day which makes you feel happier and calmer. The positive effect it has on your physical, emotional, mental, and spiritual well-being leads to a more meaningful and fulfilled life.

The ideal time to do your daily practice is in the morning before you start your day. That way, the rest of your day will be in a good mood and you can even be more productive at work. There are so many daily practices you can enjoy including singing, drawing, walking, stretching, and yoga.

However, the best daily practice to maintain a happy and healthy life is hands-on self-Reiki treatment. There are plenty of ways to start your day with Reiki, you can choose what's best for you. The following are some helpful tips to guide you in practicing Reiki daily:

- Allow at least 15 minutes to start doing Reiki. If possible, do this for 30 minutes to achieve better results. You can perform this before getting out of bed in the morning, in your room, on a couch, in the local park, or in your backyard.

    o Choose a place that is comfortable and quiet so you can focus on the treatment. Using sounds can help you go back into consciousness while doing Reiki.

- Decide which part of the body to perform hands-on Reiki. The ideal areas where you can put your hands while doing Reiki healing include the heart energy center, shoulders, head, and lower abdomen. Switch your hand positions once you feel you've transferred enough energy to that body part. However, you can complete the entire Reiki practice in the same position where it's needed.

- Be mindful of your mental state while enjoying self-Reiki. Do you think about yesterday or are you in the present moment? What are the emotions that arise while you're channeling your life force energy? Are there recurring thought patterns?

  o Can you say that your thoughts are inspiring like they are based on love, peace, gratitude, and joy? Or are they based on anger, doubt, worry, or fear? Recognize your thoughts without judgments, and then let them go.

Doing hands-on self-Reiki can help you understand your feelings and thoughts while focusing on gratitude and peace instead of worry and fear.

- Observe the sensations that occur in your palm. Do you feel the warmth on your hands while doing Reiki? Notice if the temperature remains the same throughout the session. It's perfectly normal if your hands remain at the same temperature from the beginning to the end of self-Reiki. However, observe the feeling before and after the treatment. Ideally, you should feel happier and calmer.

- Breathe deeply in your lower abdomen. Breathing in your lower belly during the session can help calm your nervous system while allowing you to be in the moment. Feel it as you breathe in and soften as you breathe out.

Practice Reiki everyday to develop positive emotions such as feelings of peace and gratitude. This daily practice will also help you align with other emotional and mental conditions for you to cope with daily challenges.

With a dedicated practice of Reiki healing, you can effectively increase your wellness. Every day gives you opportunities to be healthy and happy through this self-healing technique so you can be more kind, honest, and free from anger and worries.

How to Practice Sleep-Focused Reiki

Sleeping after a Reiki treatment can help you heal and recover more effectively from an illness. Some of the benefits of a sleep-focused Reiki include a calmer and clearer mind, higher energy levels, reduced physical pain, increased self-awareness, and a mental shift towards a successful life.

If you're wondering how sleeping during a Reiki treatment can affect the results, the good news is that it's still effective and beneficial. In fact, falling asleep while doing the treatment is a sign that you're allowing your body and mind to experience deep healing.

You may receive Reiki to stabilize your emotions and thoughts, connect yourself with something greater, boost your energy, and gain extra support while recovering from an injury or illness. This will help you regain balance when your mind, body, and spirit can restore and relax.

By activating the parasympathetic nervous system, sleep-focused Reiki can regulate digestion, lower blood pressure, and slow down the heart rate. In addition, it creates a perfect environment where healing and recovery take place. When you are completely relaxed, stress-free, and grounded, that's when true healing happens.

The reason why people fall asleep when doing Reiki is that they need to. Every day, you spend most of your energy to attend to your daily needs and responsibilities with family, colleagues, and friends. A fast-paced life can burn you out physically and emotionally, hence the need for self-Reiki practice. It works by restoring your balance, revitalizing your energy, and connecting you with yourself so your day-to-day living becomes easier and more meaningful.

Now, can Reiki cure sleep-related problems such as insomnia?

Insomnia can either be a slight problem or a debilitating condition. If you're suffering from this sleep disorder, there are a lot of solutions to help reduce the symptoms including medications, cognitive behavioral therapy, and energy healing. Reiki can help restore your normal sleep pattern through regular sessions.

Basically, insomnia occurs when you can't fall asleep no matter what you do. According to health experts, adult people need at least 7 to 8 hours of sleep to be able to function properly. If you lack sleep, you're more likely to feel sluggish, depressed, irritable, or exhausted. You may also experience difficulty focusing on your tasks, putting you at risk of injury or accidental death.

One common sign that you are having insomnia is when you usually spend 30 minutes or more in trying to fall asleep every night. If you've noticed that you're barely getting any sleep on consecutive nights, you need Reiki to help you cure your insomnia.

Below are some of the most common causes of insomnia:

- Stress. Feeling stressed out because of work, medical conditions, or relationships can lead to insomnia.

- Anxiety. When you're anxious or having an anxiety attack, it will be difficult to fall asleep which often leads to serious health conditions and other sleep issues.

- Depression. Sleep disturbances and insomnia are common to people with depression.

- Certain health conditions. Chronic pain is one of the major causes of insomnia, which often makes it hard to stay asleep.

- Environment changes. If there are recent changes to your living arrangements and schedules, this can trigger restlessness and sleep disorders.

- Poor sleep patterns. If you feel uncomfortable in your sleeping environment, you are likely to develop irregular sleep patterns.

- Too much nicotine, caffeine, or alcohol. Nicotine and caffeine are stimulants, meaning they can disturb your sleep and make it hard to fall asleep. On the other hand, alcohol is a sedative that can put your to sleep but you still won't get the rest you need if you're too drunk.

- Medications. Not all, but certain medications like corticosteroids can cause insomnia.

Knowing the causes of your insomnia can help determine the best solution to cure it. Reiki can address these problems, especially stress, anxiety, and depression. However, regardless of what's causing you to suffer from sleep issues, Reiki treatment can be beneficial. For instance, Reiki can help distribute life force energy to the parts of the body where it's needed.

If the insomnia is caused by depression, anxiety, or stress, Reiki healing can alleviate the symptoms through the following ways:

- Reiki helps you relax, so you can acknowledge your problems and put them in perspective. It will guide you in finding a spiritual and mental balance to calm the mind and fall asleep. By reducing your anxiety and stress, you can relieve the symptoms of insomnia.

- Reiki gives you self-control. If you're suffering from depression, anxiety, or stress, it's normal to feel out of control. By receiving Reiki, you can gain control of your life again. This can improve the symptoms and help you fall asleep when you need to.

- Reiki supports interpersonal relationships. During the Reiki session, you will feel that you're connected and supported by the practitioner. Reiki masters are trained to be professional and caring, so it's not surprising if you immediately feel connected with them. This interpersonal relationship can reduce the symptoms of mental problems such as depression.

Insomnia is often experienced because of certain factors that contribute to the condition. Anxiety, depression, and stress are only some of the most common factors that Reiki helps address and heal. Receiving Reiki is one of the best alternatives to relieve stress, restore your inner balance, and calm your nerves so you can sleep better.

Practicing Reiki to Relieve Stress

Living in a fast-paced world can take a toll on your physical, mental, and emotional health. It's important to learn how to adapt to the changes in your life, so you can avoid suppressed emotions that can lead to stress. Unreleased stress can lead to physical and mental diseases.

Reiki can support you daily by helping you relax and relieve stress, worry, and anxiety. This strengthens your personal power and self-esteem while encouraging you to improve your diet, exercise more, devote time to leisure activities, and avoid alcohol and tobacco.

There are different ways to practice Reiki for stress relief, below are some of the most helpful techniques:

- Usui Reiki. This traditional energy healing method doesn't require any pressure on the body during the treatment. You can lie down on the bed or sit on your couch while doing this healing technique. After the session, you will feel more relaxed and healed from stress and other negative emotions.

- Angelic Reiki. This modern way of receiving Reiki needs the healing power of ascended masters and archangels. However, you don't have to believe in them to successfully benefit from the treatment. The advantage of having faith in these supreme beings is that you become more open to the Reiki energy you receive.

While stress is normal in day to day life, it won't do you any good when prolonged. Some common sources of stress include having financial problems, running late with bad traffic, doing all the responsibilities in the family, and working for longer hours. Feeling stressed for a longer period can create imbalances in your physical, mental, and emotional health.

You have the choice to remove yourself from a stressful environment or eliminate the stressors from your life. Unfortunately, it is not that simple. You need to manage stress by exerting a lot of effort such as exercising regularly and practicing Reiki everyday.

When doing a Reiki session, certain parts of the body are focused on by practitioners. The head holds most of the stress and tension in your body, the heart stores your emotional memories, the solar plexus and stomach also hold worries and tensions, and the underbelly keeps other negative emotions and pressures.

You create harmony and balance by allowing life force energy to flow through the essential parts of your body: head, heart, solar plexus, stomach, and lower abdomen. It helps you become aware of your body and emotions while signaling you when your stress level is high.

Since Reiki works like meditation, you can consciously connect and release all emotions that are no longer beneficial to you. If you still don't believe that this method works, remember that you're made up of energy. Here's a 5-minute exercise you can do right now to relieve stress:

1. Lie down on your bed and relax.

2. Place both of your hands at the back of your head. Your palms should cradle the rear part of the skull. Do this for two minutes.

3. After the two minutes, breathe deeply while imagining your hands are transporting healing energy to your body. Release any thoughts and energies that are no longer beneficial to you. Fill your mind with calm thoughts, light, and peace for you to achieve deep relaxation. Once you are relaxed, put your hands on your chest.

4. While holding your chest, allow the energy to penetrate through your heart. Notice how your heart releases the stress, pain, undue burden, and all the heaviness that you've been keeping for some time now. Slowly release the light and energy from your hands for you to heal your heart.

5. While opening your eyes, see how your body and mind welcome the energy. The whole exercise should

make you feel light and easy, free from all the stress and worries you have before doing Reiki.

If you recently experienced mental struggles and an overactive mind, Reiki can help you release all the emotional burden you've been carrying for the past few days. Over time, this alternative healing treatment has become more widely recognized as a form of natural healing.

Reiki is generally safe and effective in relieving stress, restoring balance and wellness, and creating positive energy to heal the body. It's important to do Reiki with a certified practitioner to get the best results.

Chapter 4 - Cleansing Aura and Self-Healing Techniques

Reiki Healing Techniques to Master

Reiki healing is a very simple practice, but it is also a very powerful technique you can master. After learning the basic level, it's time to advance to the Master Level – Level II of Reiki healing. In this stage, you might find it difficult to concentrate on a deeper level. However, if you give it enough time, you will eventually get the hang of it.

Mastering the art of Reiki only requires "you". Unlike other healing treatments, Reiki doesn't have to be complicated. There's no need for sage or incense, but it's okay if you want to use them during the session. Keep in mind that it's a skill you need to learn. And everything lies in your hands, how you manage the flow of energy to achieve results.

In case you feel you're not ready to do it, you can always try again some other time. Just like learning how to ride a bike, Reiki also needs you to be patient. Learning a new skill, after all, requires time and patience. So if you're having a hard time mastering this healing technique, take a rest and try again when you're ready.

While it takes a while before learning to practice Reiki, here are some tips to make the experience easier and successful:

- Take it easy. No matter what you are trying to learn, the best way to get results is to start small. Don't pressure yourself, especially on the first day of learning. If you're not physically and mentally prepared, then you can practice the next day, or week, or month – whenever you're ready.

    o Instead of 45 minutes, you can allocate at least 10 minutes to practice Reiki. Over time, you will get used to it and practice longer once you've mastered this skill. From 10 minutes, it will eventually become 20 minutes, 30 minutes, 40 minutes, until it becomes 45 minutes.

- Make it a daily habit. Consistency is key in mastering Reiki healing. Brief and consistent sessions conducted on a daily basis can produce better results compared to long, irregular sessions. Set a schedule for your daily Reiki sessions for you to stay consistent.

    o Likewise, you may also set a specific place for your practice such as in front of an altar, on a chair, or simply on a mat to develop this habit more effectively. Placing a mat or a chair in same exact place will also encourage you to do your session. When place, time of day, and circumstances remain the same every day, it can make Reiki learning much easier and successful.

- Know your why. It's important to understand why you want to master Reiki healing. Perhaps, you want to get the most benefits out of this natural treatment including peace, clarity, inner joy, laughter, or overall wellness.

  The calming effects of energy healing bring different sensations to the body while mental thoughts and feelings are significantly changed after practicing Reiki. Do you feel calmer, more loving, open, connected, or grounded. So, why do you want to do this?

- Know your growing pains. As you age, it's normal to have problems. You don't need to punish yourself for the failures and mistakes you have committed. What matters is that you are doing what you can for you to grow and learn.

  - Once you've mastered Reiki, everything will change. Initially, you will feel a bit different because you have let go of the physical and emotional pains you've been keeping for quite some time now. Healing starts in knowing that you have it in you, that you can do it despite the struggles.

- Get a guide. A well-guided Reiki practice is the best way to learn and master this healing technique. Sometimes, it's hard to focus even if you sit down in silence. Doing a guided Reiki session will assist you through each hand position.

  - o Set your timer for 3 to 5 minutes for each position so you'll know when it's time to proceed to the next hand position. You can also use symbol mantras for each chakra, this will help you focus more while channeling your life force energy.

- Manage your expectations. What are you expecting from your Reiki training? Do you feel it's a failure when you don't achieve a certain emotion after the session? Oftentimes, people believe that they need to have certain feelings while receiving a Reiki. Others think that their mind should be clear of anything.

- o In reality, you won't instantly feel happy or free from all negative thoughts after 10 minutes of the treatment. Remember, it's a healing process wherein it takes time to produce the desired results. This practice will make you experience certain thoughts and emotions while allowing you to feel what you need to feel.

- Interrupt negative thoughts. When you notice negative thoughts clouding up your mind, use "but" for you to interrupt them. For example, if you're thinking that you're not good at Reiki, quickly interrupt it with "but, I'll get better if I continue practicing." If you're not feeling any emotions, it means it's not important. Trust the process and it will give you successful results when you're ready.

If ever you stop practicing Reiki, then start again. Always believe in yourself, that you can do anything. The success of your training lies in a positive mind, the rest will follow and fall into place. Most importantly, keep in mind that the main purpose of practicing Reiki is to be better in "being".

How to Do Self-Healing at Home

Physical and emotional well-being can be achieved through simple Reiki techniques. One of the most common exercises to do self-healing at home is a Reiki bath. This full-body overhaul helps clear stagnancies and blockages in your energy channels.

Self-care practices are essential in easing anxiety and other negative energies. You need to feel calm for you to get better sleep. In addition, a code of practice will guide you in living mindfully and positively.

Mindfulness and meditation techniques increase your Reiki energy while building a connection with your inner self.

You can try the following healing techniques that are easily doable at home:

- Take a Reiki bath. Indulging in a full-body treatment helps deepen the energy healing experience. It will help you understand your mind and body even more intuitively through the in-flow of energy during the session. Once you have performed the grounding meditation, place your hands on the energy center for 3 to 5 minutes.

  Start from your Crown chakra, then finish it on your Root chakra. Reiki bath involves similar hand positions when doing a full Reiki treatment. As you lay down in a soothing warm bath, your sensory is heightened. You can play some relaxing music, use healing crystals, or lit some scented candles to increase relaxation.

- Create a meditation sanctuary. Whether you're simply relaxing through meditation or healing with a Reiki treatment, creating a space that is exclusively for this daily practice is essential. Your sanctuary should always be ready to help you achieve self-healing whenever you need to release stress and tensions.

- Do some grounding meditation. Grounding is helpful when you're feeling unbalanced. After meditating, do this exercise for you to help you come back to your sensory so you will feel grounded. Tune in your psychic abilities to fully develop your connection with the earth. Every morning, spend 5 to 10 minutes of grounding meditation before starting your day.

Developing a consistent practice of Reiki helps ground your body so it will feel focused and clear. Breathe into your belly to experience energy healing while your life force energy supports your body, mind, and spirit. Breathe in deeply into your belly and verbalize "breathing in". When you breathe out, exhale stagnant energies and verbalize "breathing out".

Imagine yourself rooted to the ground like there's a string that is connected from your belly to the earth. Feel the grounding experience and be in the moment to heal yourself. Breathe deeply into your belly, then breathe out. Press your hands together in front of your chest and gently open your eyes.

- Journal your Reiki training. By keeping track of your practice, you can see if Reiki is really working for you. It will give you an idea of how the meditation, sensory experiences, feelings, and thoughts are affecting your body, mind, and soul. Do this everyday for you to know your progress and see which areas you can improve or benefit you the most.

- Live by the Reiki principles. Practicing the principles of Reiki in your day to day life will help you focus more on what's essential. Silently chant this, "Today, I will not anger, I will not worry, I will work with diligence, I will be kind to myself and others, and I will be grateful." Make sure to incorporate this in your meditation practice to get more relaxed and focused.

  These principles are the real essence of doing Reiki. You need to forget the past, set aside the future, and focus on the present. Connect with high vibrations of kindness and gratitude for you to benefit and support your life as well as the people around you.

Before you begin your practice, keep in mind that Reiki already exists in you. This universal life force energy only needs to be strengthened by Reiki for you to help the body heal from negative thoughts, feelings, and emotions. By practicing this natural healing treatment daily, you can become more peaceful and calmer, two things that are important in staying healthy and happy.

Illnesses That Reiki Can Help With

Reiki doesn't work like magic, it won't give you results overnight. If you have serious health problems, don't expect that they will be cured in an instant. This energy healing method only works by calming your mind, body, and spirit so your life for energy can help release suppressed tensions and negative energies in your body. If you're in a relaxed state, it's more manageable to treat your illnesses.

The following are the most common health issues that Reiki can help with:

- Pain

- Nausea

- Sleep problems

- Brain disorders

- Infertility

- Chronic fatigue syndrome

- Cancer

Now, let's focus on Parkinson's disease.

Despite the lack of study in the advantages of Reiki for patients with Parkinson's, some researchers found out that this natural treatment can somehow relieve pain and depression. Many people are practicing this technique to trigger positive thinking and feelings of calm, well-being, and being in control of your body, mind, and spirit.

Here's how Reiki healing addresses the body, mind, and soul of people with Parkinson's and other brain disorders:

- Reiki energy nourishes the body and heals damaged tissues. It also promotes detoxifying and natural healing of the body by releasing energy blockages.

- Reiki meditation calms and relaxes your mind by relieving stress and balancing your emotions and thoughts.

- The life force energy that is channeled through Reiki connects with your spirit. Therefore, it nourishes and heals you on a deeper level.

According to Reiki masters, this energy healing method has potential benefits for those who are suffering from Parkinson's. For instance, it helps regulate the area in the brain which releases dopamine. Also, it improves the functioning of the barrier between blood and brain for you to support the delivery of medication to the brain in a more efficient way.

The natural healing ability and vitality of the body is also improved after a Reiki session. It channels the life force energy to the organs that are hugely affected by the medications that treat the symptoms of

Parkinson's disease. However, it's important to understand that the response of every patient to the treatment will be different.

Before you decide to undergo Reiki treatment, it's highly recommended to consult your doctor. You can also seek advice from those who have personal experiences doing Reiki for their Parkinson's, such as your family, friends, and the local community. More importantly, get a Reiki practitioner who has firsthand experience healing patients with this kind of brain disorder.

Studies on using Reiki to help with cancer patients are also becoming more widely recognized. A study conducted in Canada showed that cancer patients who were given Reiki treatments experienced less pain after the sessions. One of the most common symptoms of cancer is pain, Reiki can help reduce this while giving the patient a relaxed and peaceful mind.

However, some people experienced headaches, weakness, tiredness, and stomach upset after receiving Reiki treatment. If you also experience these symptoms, that means your body is getting rid of toxins. The best way to treat these symptoms is to eat lighter meals, drink more water, and take a rest.

In the case of autoimmune diseases, Reiki treatment can also help manage the symptoms and improve the quality of life. The most common types of autoimmune illnesses include celiac disease, multiple sclerosis, type I diabetes, rheumatoid arthritis, and Grave's disease.

The following are the benefits of using Reiki on patients with autoimmune diseases:

- Pain reduction. Pain is a debilitating symptom of patients with autoimmune diseases such as multiple sclerosis and rheumatoid arthritis. They experience chronic pain but claim that the pain sensations are reduced after receiving Reiki treatment.

- Emotional and physical balance improvement. Many Reiki clients claim that the treatment improved their emotional and physical balance. As a result, they can manage chronic illnesses in a much better way which improves their quality of life.

- Depression and anxiety management. Depression and anxiety are common among people who are suffering from autoimmune diseases due to painful symptoms. Receiving Reiki can help decrease anxiety and improve your mood. Once your mind, body, and spirit are harmonized and balanced, it offers great benefits to your overall condition.

- Stronger immunity. By doing Reiki regularly, patients experience less painful symptoms of their autoimmune diseases. Also, this alternative healing treatment offers a low risk of side effects since it's non-invasive, natural, and painless.

More people are recognizing the benefits of this energy healing technique, especially its valuable role in providing alternative options for those who can't afford expensive medical procedures.

According to Modern Physics, the energy fields in your body flow through glands, organs, and cells to nourish them. Any imbalances in your energy field can make you vulnerable to diseases. The unstable flow of energy also manifests infection, stress, and other discomforts that can be felt emotionally, mentally, or physically. If you have chronic illnesses, it can conversely affect your body by creating imbalances in your energy fields.

How to Cleanse Your Aura

Basically, your aura refers to the energy flow within your body and around you. It flows and radiates from you while absorbing all sorts of energies including negative energy around you. Once it's full of bad energy, your aura becomes foggy. You will feel heavy and weak, making it difficult to concentrate on what you need to do.

It's important to cleanse your aura regularly because humans are sensitive beings and energy is highly contagious. That means you can easily pick up certain energies and feelings from other people after interacting with them. You can absorb negative energy and feel sick due to emotional issues and intuition blockages.

Auras are energetic fields surrounding the body, hence representing current vibrations and emotions. Your aura can reveal what's in your heart and mind as well as your desires. Therefore, you need to take care of your aura for you to stay healthy and happy.

Aside from bad energy, there are other negative things that can dull your aura. For instance, stress is one of the most common causes of drained energy. It's important to protect your aura from all negativity for you to stay physically, mentally, and spiritually healthy.

The following are simple techniques to cleanse and protect your aura:

- Take a shower or soak in the bathtub to get rid of negative energies. This will help you feel refreshed after immersing your body in the bathtub. The best way to do this aura cleansing is to use essential oils, sacred herbs, and salts to clear the energy fields.

  - Fill your bathtub with water and then add Himalayan salt and lavender or any essential oils to increase the cleansing effects. You can soak yourself for 10 minutes or more depending on how much negative energy you need to cleanse. If you're taking shower, imagine your aura being healed and cleansed while the water flows down through your feet.

- Burn some sacred herbs like sage. Smudging is an old aura cleansing technique that still works today. You can use dried white sage to cleanse your aura and get rid of bad vibes. Other sacred herbs you can use include cedar and thyme. Burn the bundles just like what you do in incense sticks, then allow the smoke to be absorbed by your body.

- Enjoy the rain. Walking in the rain is an easy way to clean your aura. When it rains outside, go out and feel the raindrops on your skin while your eyes are closed. Visualize the rain washing away the toxic energy in your body.

    o If it's not raining in your area, you can go swimming in a nearby lake as it has the same effects on your energy fields. Water is an essential element in clearing your mind, body, and spirit of negative energies. However, don't walk in the rain if there are thunderstorms.

- Do the combing exercise. Before you do this aura cleansing exercise, make sure you washed your hands. Find an area in your house that is quiet and comfortable. Visualize your aura while your eyes are closed, then start combing your head down to your toes.

  o It's important to constantly visualize the energy as your aura is getting cleaned with every comb. After doing this exercise, wash your hands again to rinse off the bad energy.

- Recite your affirmations and mantras. Another effective method to cleanse your aura is to sit quietly and imagine yourself with an effervescent light surrounding you. Start chanting positive affirmations and mantras while your eyes are closed.

Recite the affirmations several times until the message vibrates through your physical body.

You can practice this everyday to fortify your energy fields.

The next time you fall sick and feel wound up and irritated, clear your energy channels from any blockages to feel relaxed and calm. A clear aura helps you sleep better and think more clearly without distractions and negative thoughts.

A stressed or weak aura also affects your quality of life, especially your relationships with family and friends. The auric field is susceptible to stress because you consistently exchange energies with every person you come across. For you to avoid feeling impatient, lethargic, irritated, anxious, or stressed, make sure to regularly cleanse your aura with these simple exercises.

By keeping your aura in a positive state, you can boost your immune system while being able to heal from chronic pain and other symptoms of stress. You can do cleansing aura techniques in your home to promote better focus and energy flow.

Here are the colors of the aura and their meanings:

- Black – change and transformation.

- Brown – greed and selfishness.

- Grey – exhaustion and sadness.

- White – balance and harmony.

- Pink – kindness and gentleness.

- Violet – psychic and spiritual.

- Indigo – clairvoyant and intuitive.

- Blue – sensitive and artistic.

- Green – peaceful and compassionate.

- Yellow – happiness and positivity.

- Orange – valor and willfulness.

- Red – exuberance and passion.

If there are different colors reflecting your aura, that means you have different energies flowing within you. However, the combination of colors that indicate you are effectively cleansing your aura are brown, black, and grey. So if you meet someone with negative energy, it's best to do the cleansing aura exercises to prevent exhausting your energy. Avoid people with an evil eye, those who love to gossip, and people who are always jealous.

Chapter 5 - Reiki and Nutrition

How to Use Reiki in Boosting Food Energy

You might think that Reiki is only for healing and calming the mind, body, and spirit. Practicing this energy healing technique has a lot of benefits to your health, but you can also use it to boost your food. Every person and object such as food should be secured with life force energy for you to keep them protected from harm.

The majority of food products available today are factory-made and not fresh. If you eat processed foods every day, it can be toxic to your body. The accumulated "poison" will weaken your life force energy and lead to health problems in the future. This is why it's important to use Reiki on your food to ensure it doesn't have energetic impurities that can cause diseases.

According to macrobiotics, food is spirit. There's a connection between the food you eat and the effects it has on your body, mind, and spirit. You can grow your own food, prepare your everyday meals, and eat natural food as part of your spiritual practices.

So how do you use Reiki on your food?

If you feel unsatisfied or don't have enough energy even after you eat, your food might be lacking in Ki or life force energy. This non-physical energy is responsible for giving life to every living thing. It should be strong and free to flow through your body to boost your well-being and other important aspects of life.

It's important to receive and practice Reiki to boost your energy and overall health. Understanding the relationship of Ki with the food you eat is a good starting point to realize the benefits of boosting your food with Reiki. You see, food is not just about vitamins, minerals, fat, carbohydrates, and protein.

If you want to receive Ki daily, you can do that by eating healthy foods including fresh vegetables and fruits. These foods have higher Ki content than processed foods and other unhealthy products. Below are the easiest ways to practice Reiki in boosting your food:

- Grow your own garden. If you're a gardener, you can use Reiki on your herbs and vegetables. They actually love receiving Ki energy as it helps them grow healthier. Give them their daily dose of Reiki and expect higher yields.

- Use Reiki when you cook and prepare food at home. Put the ingredients on your hands and channel Ki energy into them. You can also place your hands over the food to bless it with positive energy before eating. The intention is to eliminate the negative effects of eating the food, and rather increased the positive benefits to the body.

o Always start with eliminating the negative before working on to boost the positive effects of the food. You can visualize or draw the emotional symbol over your food, then follow it with the power symbol to strengthen the universal energy. Do this regularly when you prepare food for your loved ones to help them enjoy the food while boosting their health.

- Add Ki energy to your meals. Before you eat, make it a habit to Reiki your food. Hold your hands over the plate to channel the energy while getting rid of negative energy from your food. You can imagine or draw the emotional and power symbols over the food. Always bless your food with positive energy to enjoy your meals and eat healthily.

- Energize your food when eating in a restaurant. If you're eating out, it's also effective to use Reiki. This helps to clear and charge the food since you're not sure how it was prepared. Sometimes the person serving your food is in a bad mood, their negative energy can be absorbed by your body. Put your palms under the table and point your fingers up at the food to transfer positive energy.

Reiki raises the vibrations of the food including grains, fruits, vegetables, and animal products. You can also use the distance symbol for you to connect with devas and angels to secure the food you're going to eat is pure and healthy. If you're unpacking your groceries, Reiki them as well so that the Divine and Mother Earth will restore their energy and eliminate toxins.

It's not enough to use Reiki in healing your mind, body, and spirit. You should also do this technique to boost your food for you to get more nutrition and satisfaction from what you're eating every single day.

<u>Why Ki Is Essential in the Food You Eat</u>

Your diet should be exciting and pleasurable rather than plain and bland. It's essential to fill your plate with colorful veggies and fruits that add life to your meals. However, if you really want to get the most benefits out of your daily food, you can use Reiki to boost nutrients and make it more appetizing.

By learning how you can combine nutrition, energy healing, and modern science for you to achieve overall wellness, you will understand the best practices to get results. With a holistic approach to self-healing, you can surely enjoy your everyday meals while boosting their nutrition through Ki energy.

So, why do you need to perform Reiki treatment on your food?

Your goal should be to live healthily so that your existence radiates inner truth, positive thoughts, a healthy body, peaceful spirit, good intuition, a loving heart, and inspiring emotions. According to science, your food choices can affect your mood. Therefore, you need to be smart in choosing what you include in your diet as well as how to increase Ki energy so you can harmonize and balance your body, mind, and spirit.

If you think you're eating a diet that lacks nutrition, it's important to eliminate unhealthy food choices starting today. You may be packing in foods that contain empty calories, this will only lead to unhealthy weight and other health issues. So as early as now, you need to focus on the essential foods that provide the vitamins and minerals your body needs.

For instance, eating elderberries, dates, and quince can affect your mood. Boosting Ki in these foods can help you create positive mood that is essential in living a happy and meaningful life. In addition, you can eat chicory and lettuce as natural tranquilizers while eggs, beef, pomegranates, and apples serve as sensual stimulants.

A modern lifestyle involves some health challenges, making it a bit hard to maintain and improve your health in the long run. The food you eat has a huge impact on the quality of your life, your weight, mood, appearance, and energy. By using Reiki on your food, it can help enhance your life force energy which leads to positive thinking, vigor, rejuvenation, and optimal health.

Moreover, Reiki treated food gives you the power to heal from stress, depression, chronic pain, and other ailments that are affecting your body, mind, and spirit. You can use salt and sugar in moderation while preparing Reiki food for you to promote self-healing.

Reiki energized food will help you harmonize and balance your emotions as it aligns the chakras in your body, hence increasing your optimism. Charge your salt and sugar with environmental energies including Reiki, Music, Quartz Crystals, and Pyramid for you to energize your body through energy channels while soothing your nerves and relaxing your mind.

Quartz Crystals and Music help synchronize your chakras to boost healing and bring out wellness and balance. However, Reiki is the best way to improve your healing power and enhance your entire being. The following are some helpful tips to boost Ki energy in what you eat:

- Don't eat too much at night. Eat your dinner 3 hours before bedtime.

- Never skip your breakfast as it can trigger mood swings and anxiety.

- Chew slowly for you to help your body digest food and boost immunity.

- You should be in a good mood when preparing your meals so that you can transfer positive energy to your food.

When your chakras are balanced and energized with Ki, you will experience the following:

- Feel and understand your body.

- Honor your emotions.

- Maintain alignment and balance between your work and life.

- Embrace self-love and care for others.

- Speak the truth more compassionately.

- Tune in to your intuition.

- Lead a meaningful and purposeful life.

Aside from eating healthy foods, you also need to focus on drinking plenty of water to maintain good digestion. Also, water helps keep things moving in your body including the flow of energy. The flow should help with your emotions and eating practices so that you can reduce unhealthy food cravings that can affect your health.

Perform a 7-day Reiki Food program to concentrate on your health system. Within one week, apply Ki energy to your food, water, and other items that you take in your body. This will help you reduce physical symptoms including poor sleep, pain, and fatigue. Food Reiki is also important in dealing with mental and emotional issues including emotional eating, perfectionism, and overthinking.

Your internal environment reflects your external surroundings. Therefore, restoring your body and mind wellness lies in your inner self; what's enveloping you, how you're dealing with people, and what you're eating.

What to Do If You Forgot to Reiki Your Food

If your food contains a lower level of Ki, you might feel depleted after you eat rather than feel replenished. One of the most common reasons foods don't have enough life force energy is that they are contaminated with pesticides while others are grown in areas where air quality is poor.

Moreover, some animal products may still contain the energy of animals. For meat products, they may store the fear or anger of animals while being slaughtered.

This is the main reason why Reiki masters don't recommend eating animal products.

How your food is handled also affects the Ki, such as climate conditions, irritated workers, and angry servers in a restaurant. Imagine the things your food need to pass through from its origin to your table, they all affect the life force energy in the food. So basically, how the food is transported can reduce Ki levels especially if your food will take weeks before it reaches your plate.

How the food is prepared and cooked also affects the energy it contains. Some cooking methods can even destroy Ki including microwaving, freezing, and boiling. Good thing you can raise the level of Ki in your food to get the most health benefits after eating.

Food is efficient in storing life force energy, making it a vital source of energy. Therefore, it's important to do Reiki on your food before consuming them for you to ensure that you are getting the right amount of energy your body needs to function properly. With a daily practice of Reiki, you can increase the level of life force energy while eliminating detrimental energies the food may contain.

Now, what if you forget to charge and cleanse your food?

There's no need to worry about forgetting to Reiki the meal you have just consumed. Simply put your palms on your belly after eating to charge it with Ki energy. You can practice this every mealtime to cleanse the food you are about to it. Also, Reiki treatment after eating can help soothe your stomach especially if you have eaten too much food.

In addition, this energy healing technique can help with digestion and improve the absorption of nutrients in your body. Remember, the digestion process will take more energy than other major bodily functions. If your food is digested more easily and faster, there will be more energy for you to consume during physical activities.

Digesting food efficiently also give you more energy than simply letting it sit in your intestine for a longer period which only contribute to toxicity in your body. For you to feel replenished and energized after eating, make sure you do Reiki on your food. If you forgot, you can just do the energy charging on your stomach by placing your hands and visualizing Reiki symbols.

But what if you don't practice this healing technique daily, or at all?

Every day, your body requires sufficient energy to function and fight off illnesses. If you don't Reiki your food before you eat, it might not be efficient in giving you the energy you need as well as the vitamins and minerals needed to protect you from bacteria and viruses.

There are so many options you can do to make sure you are eating healthy foods daily. For example, hand positions can help you boost Ki levels in your food and clear off negative energies that may block the flow of energy through your chakras and energy channels. Recite your intention while holding your hands on your stomach or over the food you are going to eat.

Imagine a white light surrounding your hands and intend it to cleanse your body from bad energies. Then begin to charge and fill the food with life force energy for you to get the health benefits you need.

If you have issues with your relationship with food such as eating disorders, it's important to practice Reiki healing so that you can improve your mind, body, and spirit through the food you eat. During the session, say that you honor your entire body and accept the nourishment into your being.

Eventually, you will notice that eating is becoming less focused on internal power struggles, guilt, and fear. Instead, you slowly realize that it is more on the energy you receive that helps improve the quality of your life physically, mentally, and spiritually.

You are what you eat. So make sure you are filling yourself with more Ki energy than the usual amount you get from typical cooking and food preparation methods. Once you embrace the importance of Reiki treatment in your daily diet, it's easy to feel how your energy levels increase while your overall health becomes more stable.

The Power of Reiki Food Therapy

Have you experienced feeling sickness or pressure in your abdominal area after having an argument with someone? Perhaps you've lost your appetite while grieving the loss of a loved one. Emotions can lessen the flow of blood through your body while stress puts your immune system at risk of illnesses and infections.

Reiki food therapy helps heal the body, mind, and soul. It boosts nourishment and quality of life while slowing down the aging process. Everyone knows that food is essential in building the body, but only a few are aware of the importance of self-healing for you to maintain a positive mind, healthy body, and a compassionate soul.

Eating energy-charged food has a direct effect on your body, mind, and spirit. But what does Reiki food therapy really mean?

Reiki food therapy refers to a method wherein the food is charged with environmental energies for you to harmonize and balance your emotions and align your chakras. By doing so, you can increase your positivity in life while energizing your body with life force energy.

Everything around you including animals, plants, and non-living things has their own energy frequency. Sending Reiki to your food can help enhance its energy while reducing any potential negative energies. This is really important because people tend to indulge in unhealthy foods such as fast food and other processed foods.

By boosting Reiki in your food, you can get more nutritional value from what you eat. In Japan, this is a very common practice which obviously explains why Japanese people are healthier and live longer than other nationalities. They also believe that Reiki treatment helps make your food taste better and purer. Normally, you do this before eating for you to take in positive energy from the food.

There might not be an exact diet that can cure migraines or clinical depression, but just by being aware of the food you consume and treating it with Reiki can help give you amazing results. Having a positive mind and a strong immune system will help you feel great. However, make sure to practice avoiding stress and anger for you to boost your Ki energy in the body.

For instance, never skip your breakfast because it will only increase your anxiety and can make you feel irritated the entire day. Also, it's important to eat less at night to help recharge your body and wake up feeling blissful and blessed in the morning.

Mindful eating is essential in building strong immunity which has a big impact on your overall health. Optimism and a good mood while cooking helps transfer higher levels of Ki into your food. Remember, our modern lifestyles come with new challenges in terms of maintaining and improving wellness and well-being. Therefore, you really have to step up your self-healing abilities through the daily practice of Reiki treatment.

Below is a simple recipe for an organic bean meal from Rose Elliot's Vegetarian Fast Food. You can easily prepare this at home and do Reiki to boost its nutrients:

Ingredients:

Olive oil – 1 tablespoon

Onion – 1 piece, chopped

Baked beans – 1 can

Red kidney beans – 15 ounces, drained

Corn kernels – 1 cup, drained

Bread – 4-6 slices

Nonfat Cheddar cheese – 1 cup, grated

Instructions:

1. Pour the olive oil in your saucepan and heat. Add the chopped onions, cook, and cover it for 10 minutes. Check if it's softened, then add the corn, kidney beans, and baked beans. Cook everything together and gently stir until it's hot.

2. Pour the cooked mixture into a heatproof dish. Add some bread slices on top of the beans and finish it with grated Cheddar cheese.

3. Put the dish in a heated broiler and broil it for 5 minutes until the cheese has melted and the bread pieces are crisp and golden brown.

4. Serve right away. This recipe is good for up to 4 servings.

One serving may contain 465 calories, 1,756 milligrams of sodium, 5 milligrams of cholesterol, 83 grams of carbohydrates, 26 grams of protein, and 6.3 grams of fat.

To boost Reiki in your baked beans, place your hands over the bowl and visualize the Power symbol or any symbols you want to use. Blessing your food before eating is an essential practice to get more from what you eat daily. Do this healing technique even in the simplest meal you have prepared to ensure you are getting high energies that your body, mind, and soul need.

Chapter 6 - Interesting Facts About Reiki

Who is Mikao Usui Sensei?

For you to understand Reiki on a deeper level, it's important to get to know the father of this natural healing practice – Dr. Mikao Usui, also known as the Usui Sensei.

The Usui Sensei was the founder of Reiki healing which originated in Japan. He was born on August 15, 1865, to an affluent Buddhist family. As a notable Tendai Buddhist at the time, Dr. Mikao was very fortunate to live for 11 generations in Yamagata.

At a young age of 4, he was sent to study in the Buddhist monastery. He learned swordsmanship, Kiko, or the Japanese version of Chi Kung, and martial arts. To add to his credentials, Dr. Mikao also studied theology, psychology, and medicine which led him to the discovery of a self-healing method through a hands-on approach.

However, his interest in finding a way to heal himself was not connected to any religious beliefs or religion. Therefore, Dr. Mikao's Reiki healing is accessible to anyone who needs to realign their life force energy and harmonize their body, mind, and spirit.

Before the time when Japan isolated itself from the Western world, Dr. Mikao was able to visit China, America, and Europe where he learned about the Western civilizations and cultures. During his higher education years, he learned Sanskrit, Chinese, and English and was believed to be fluent in these languages that he became a Japanese literature doctor.

Dr. Mikao had taken different professions during his time that included jobs as a missionary, office worker, reporter, Postmaster General, and Private Secretary to name a few. Later on, he got married to Sadako Suzuki, had two kids named Toshiko and Fuji, and lived a happy life. He had three siblings named Kuniji who was a policeman, Sanya who was a doctor, and sister Tsuru.

In case you're interested in visiting the remains of the Usui Sensei, the ashes of the whole family were buried in Kyoto's famous Saihoji Temple.

Now, how did Dr. Mikao discover energy healing? His spiritual path will explain everything.

In the 1900s, Dr. Mikao almost died of an illness in the middle of an epidemic. This near-death experience changed his life and pushed him to reflect on what really matters. After his recovery, he started researching on deep Buddhist healing and asked for mentorship from spiritual healers.

After seeing great potential in him, a priest accepted to teach him and Dr. Mikao then became a Shingon Buddhist. Unfortunately, this led to a big turn of events. His family banished him because they did not approve of the new life that Dr. Mikao wants to lead. However, this didn't stop him from pursuing the life he dreamed of. And so he fulfilled his dream and tread the higher spiritual path.

With the advice and guidance of fellow monks and his teacher, Dr. Mikao decided to go on a pilgrimage in Mount Kurama where Japanese people usually do spiritual quests. For 21 days, he stayed in the mountain to achieve enlightenment or Satori. To prepare for the quest, he did fasting, prayer, and meditation.

After three weeks, Dr. Mikao experienced a deep musing where he received the beam of white light glowing on the top of his head. While receiving the light, he also envisioned different Reiki symbols with spiritual guidance on how to transfer the energy through them.

That was when he felt the awakening and excitedly went down to share what he experienced in the mountain with fellow priests and his teacher. He told them that while going up the mountain, a rock hit his toe and he fell off the dirt. He put his hands over the injured toe to transfer Reiki energy. The healing energy flowed from his palms and the pain was gone.

Dr. Mikao realized that he did not only achieved enlightenment but also gained self-healing ability. This led him to an epiphany that he needs to help other people heal by teaching them Reiki since he already achieved his life purpose. He started in nearby villages until he reached Tokyo to help the needy.

As he helped people heal, he established his own healing society and called it Usui Reiki Rhoyo Gakkani which means the Usui Reiki Healing Method Society. Dr. Mikao's healing society faced a big challenge when a strong earthquake hit Yokohama and Tokyo in 1923. More than 140,000 Japanese died in the earthquake due to the fires from the massive disruption.

Together with his students, Dr. Mikao did their best to heal people who were affected by the calamity. That was when he received an award from the Emperor after healing the injured and wounded at the time. The great work he has done is still remembered up to this day.

What are the 5 Principles of Reiki?

With the success of Dr. Mikao's healing society, he opened a bigger clinic in Tokyo. It continued to give amazing results which made him even more popular across Japan. His reputation in hands-on energy healing went on and led him to initiate over 2000 students during his lifetime.

There were 20 students who became Shihan or Masters of Reiki. Cujiro Hayashi became one of the most successful students who then became a Grand Master of the healing method.

So, what are the 5 principles of Reiki that Usui Sensei developed?

There are different levels of Reiki that Dr. Mikao had developed during his time including the Shoden, Shinpiden, and Okuden. These led him to other healing techniques namely Byosen or Scanning and Gassho, a praying position.

These levels gave his students slowly but surely learning progress without flooding their minds. For you to transfer attunements to the Reiki masters, Dr. Mikao developed Reiju Kai, a more formal energy healing practice where students receive the full level of Reiki.

Emperor Meiji recommended 5 admonitions to Dr. Mikao which he later cultivated as the 5 principles of Reiki healing:

1. *Just for today, I will be grateful.* Showing gratitude for all the blessings you are receiving is important in living a good life. This principle talks about being present in your daily moments without rushing into anything.

For instance, take time to smell the flowers, bask in the sun, and feel the fresh air. Be mindful of your surroundings for you to appreciate what the Divine Power has bestowed upon us.

2. *Just for today, I will not anger.* To be angry doesn't necessarily mean you're bad. Sometimes, it only means that someone has crossed the boundaries while you can't control what others do. The important thing is to understand how you manage your anger.

If something angers you, take the time to determine the reason behind it. Then sit in silence and reflect on it before taking actions. You don't have to suppress your emotions, but you need to deal with your anger so that you can avoid whatever is triggering this intense emotion.

3. *Just for today, I will not worry.* When you tend to always worry about what's to come, your ego gets overwhelmed. You need to live in the present rather than imagining things that haven't happened yet. To help you live in the present, practice focusing on the moment.

Tap into your faith and breathe into the current moment. This can help bring you back to your consciousness and concentrate on what you need to do today. After all, worrying is a foolish act; it's like standing under an umbrella waiting for the rain.

4. *Just for today, I will do my work honestly.* One of the most rewarding goals you should strive for is to be your authentic self. It can be challenging to practice being true to yourself, but it will give you freedom no matter the circumstances. Instead of trying to fit in, always honor yourself, and don't compromise self-love for temporary acceptance from others.

Allowing your true self to shine even if others don't accept you is essential in living an optimistic life. Never hide your truth and always keep it real. So for today, make sure to focus on doing your work honestly. It may be hard at first, but taking baby steps can help you develop this good habit.

5. *Just for today, I will respect all life.* Honoring your parents, the elderly, and teachers is important in building harmonious relationships with others. You should celebrate your roots and cultivate gratitude for people who guided you when you needed it the most.

You don't have to put your parents on pedestals, a simple respect is all that you need to show gratitude.

This principle is also about growing and learning with open-mindedness and sincerity. If you show compassion and understanding toward others, it can help heal anger and judgment. In return, you can enjoy a healthy and happy life while maintaining honorable relationships with your family and friends.

The precepts that Reiki energy healing practice offers are key to a happier life while they serve as medicine to your spirit. They are like affirmations that help you focus on the present and be in the moment. The purpose of these principles is to encourage you to embody life force energy every day. Simply put, they promote the importance of being in the moment and feeling your energy from deep within.

There's no exact way to apply these principles to your daily life. You can use them during meditation or as morning affirmations. The important thing is to use them whenever it's needed such as in boosting your energy for you to attain your highest good. They will help you create balance in your body, mind, and soul while giving you spiritual attunement.

Do Studies Approve of Reiki Healing?

Before a physician or healthcare practitioner can recommend a healing practice or treatment to patients, there has to be solid evidence that it's effective and safe to use. In terms of safety, research studies haven't reported any negative effects or potential risks of Reiki healing.

It's not surprising to know that Reiki is safe because it doesn't require applying or ingesting any sort of medication for you to get results. Reiki treatment is non-manipulative, which means it can be given off the body whenever necessary. This is a non-invasive healing technique that has been used in many parts of the world for thousands of years now.

Certain measures have been studied by researchers including stress, anxiety, and pain. They also considered other primary outcomes such as caring efficacy, job burnout, salivary cortisol, blood pressure, and heart rate. These measures were used to assess results for chronic health problems, depression, and stroke rehabilitation.

With the comparatively complex and perceptive nature of energy healing, these measures and outcomes may not precisely capture the personal experiences of patients who received Reiki. On the other hand, measures that involve stress reduction, patient satisfaction, and quality of life may be more effective in proving the benefits of Reiki healing practice.

According to a randomized single-blind trial of the effectiveness of Reiki healing therapy in improving well-being and mood, students who received Reiki showed greater mood and health benefits than students who did not receive Reiki treatment. The study evaluated the impact of depression and anxiety on university students. The first 20 students are suffering from anxiety and depression while the other 20 have low anxiety and depression.

All the students received six 30-minute Reiki sessions for 8 weeks. However, they weren't aware that non-contact Reiki was given because they were absorbed in deep and guided relaxation. Researchers evaluated the effectiveness of the intercession using measures like sleep, illness symptoms, and mood.

The students with depression and anxiety who received the treatment demonstrated progressive improvements in their overall mood. On the other hand, students with low depression and anxiety showed no changes. In the conclusion of the study, Reiki healing may provides benefits to the patient's mood.

To date, Reiki has been increasingly offered in private practice settings, hospices, and hospitals for various medical conditions and illnesses. Patients who receive this energy healing treatment reported relief from health symptoms, particularly mental health problems. Many studies show that this alternative treatment primarily helps reduce stress, chronic pain, depression, and anxiety.

Although there are many studies conducted to prove the effectiveness of Reiki healing, their quality varies to a certain degree. For instance, the Center for Reiki Research examines different groups through the "touchstone process". It's an extensive peer review technique used to analyze scientific studies with the use of Reiki.

The results involve a series of critical reports from a consistent and impartial process that incorporates intensive exercises for scientific reviews. The process reevaluates every aspect of the research and how the investigations are carried out. Basically, the outcomes are analyzed while the weaknesses and strengths are observed.

Up to now, the touchstone process has already produced almost three dozens of thoroughly analyzed studies. Some conclusions drawn from the studies regarding the efficacy of Reiki healing indicated better quality or at least satisfactory. Other bodies of research show the effects of Reiki on patient's mental health. Reiki Master Joe Potter from the UK has been investigating its effectiveness to help more people understand the mental benefits of this natural healing treatment.

According to Potter's investigation, stress is the most frequent word used by patients to describe their conditions during their initial Reiki session. After the treatment, some of the clear signs produced include reduced stress as seen in the changes in heart rate and other biological measurements used.

A study conducted for nurses suffering from burnout syndrome showed some biological signals of relaxation response after undergoing Reiki treatment. Likewise, when the nurses gave Reiki to their patients suffering from acute coronary syndrome, there were reported physiological signals of relaxation effects.

While most of the scientific studies conducted on the effects of Reiki have design limitations, there is some evidence that it can really influence the recipient's mood and stimulate physiological changes both in humans and animals. Therefore, gentle touch can help produce outcomes such as pain relief and stress reduction, especially when done in a safe environment.

Is Reiki More Effective than Other Placebo Therapies?

The official website of the Center for Reiki Research has listed 70 institutions where Reiki treatment is offered. It's seen as a cost-reducing and effective method to help improve the quality of care and health outcomes. Nurses, physicians, and other hospital staff are offering Reiki due to its proven effectiveness in aiding patients including those suffering from mental health issues.

But is Reiki really more effective than a placebo?

Some experts say that placebo therapies such as Reiki may help in improving the well-being of cancer patients, but it may deprive them of other safer and more effective treatment methods.

There was an interesting study conducted by nurses in America that led to bizarre conclusions. A total of 200 cancer patients were recruited by the nurses to receive Reiki treatment despite them undergoing chemotherapy. Obviously, it's a hard time for them to try out other treatments while they're experiencing fatigue, depression, nausea, and hair loss.

Cancer symptoms decrease the quality of life and well-being of patients, therefore the nurses decided to test them for Reiki healing for you to see if it will improve their symptoms. A lot of people believe that energy healing can help reduce cancer symptoms and make life much better for anyone who has cancer. So, does Reiki really work?

A control group was used for you to find out if Reiki healing is effective. The nurses compared the results from Reiki, sham Reiki, and no intervention groups. A non-Reiki master pretended to heal the patients in the sham Reiki group. He didn't have any experience or knowledge in using Reiki healing so he just followed the Reiki practitioner's ritual. Basically, there's no healing energy transferred to the cancer patients from the sham Reiki master.

The results were impressive – Reiki treatment improved the symptoms of the patients. It increased their well-being and comfort unlike the patients from the no intervention group. However, the patients in the sham Reiki group also had the same results as the Reiki group. In other words, the sham and real Reiki did not have any differences.

The nurses concluded that Reiki did work on patients with cancer. The only problem is that real Reiki was deemed to be no better compared to sham Reiki. So, should we avoid this treatment because it's not better than other placebo therapies? Scientifically speaking, administering placebos such as Reiki may deprive cancer patients of certain treatment benefits. However, this will be for the patient to decide whether or not Reiki healing is good for them.

On a lighter note, Reiki has been proven to improve cancer patient's well-being as well as chronic symptoms. Therefore, if the patient receiving energy healing benefits from it, then healthcare professionals should be open to offering this treatment in their hospitals.

Understanding, dedication, sympathy, and empathy can go a long way to help people who are suffering from certain health problems. In addition, there's a study that says <u>Reiki is better than a placebo and has broad potential as a complementary health therapy</u>. It is said that Reiki provides more benefits and efficacy than other placebo therapies.

Out of 13 suitable peer-reviewed clinical studies, 8 concluded that Reiki is more effective and safer than placebos, 4 demonstrated no difference yet there was an alleged statistical resolving power, and one found clear evidence that there's really no benefit at all. Obviously, there's reasonable support from these studies that Reiki can benefit patients more than a placebo can provide.

This gentle and safe complementary therapy helps activate the nervous system for you to heal the mind and body. The potential effects for broader application in chronic health condition management make it even more relevant than ever before. It can also possibly aid in faster recovery from medical operations and surgeries. However, more studies are needed to prove that Reiki can really help patients manage their symptoms physically, mentally, and spiritually.

There's only one thing you need to keep in mind, Reiki isn't an alternative to cancer treatments and allopathic medicine. It's only a complementary method to achieve some level of therapeutic effects. This gentle technique is most effective in helping patients deal with depression, anxiety, and pain.

Now, what's the status of studies and research efforts made for Reiki?

While debates on the effectiveness of Reiki and other integrative therapies are gaining steam, researchers continue to study the effects and benefits of these natural healing techniques. In fact, the National Center for Complementary and Integrative Health has completed several studies about the ability of Reiki to benefit patients with fibromyalgia, prostate cancer, advanced AIDS, and diabetes.

Existing studies are not well designed and typically small, but overlapping data shows strong support to Reiki's benefits in reducing pain and anxiety. Researchers suggest this healing therapy to induce relaxation and relieve people from stress which is mainly causing other medical complications. It's not surprising that more wellness programs are offering this treatment to address burnouts and improve the skills of healthcare professionals.

Chapter 7 - Advanced Reiki Sessions:

What to Expect

What is an Advanced Usui Reiki?

Advanced Usui Reiki isn't about learning new hand positions and symbols. Rather, it is a deeper understanding of the 5 principles and applying them to your daily life. You need to trust the universal wisdom for you to guide you while performing hands-on healing.

According to Usui Sensei, *this is surely a secret process to bring a good fortune and also a miraculous medicine to remedy all kinds of diseases.* Only positive outcomes are aimed by the styles of advanced Reiki for you to honor the core essence of Usui Sensei's original healing art or spiritual practice.

Usui Reiki refers to the source of universal energy which works like gravity. If you take a step off a ledge, you will automatically fall as gravity pulls you down. The impact and speed of your fall will depend on your weight and the height of the ledge from the ground.

Throwing a ball or any object into the air will also end up in the ball hitting the ground without doing or saying anything. What does this mean when it comes to practicing Usui Reiki? Once your pathway is cleared by a Usui Reiki master and you take the time to learn and practice Usui Reiki exercises, the universal energy will flow through you even without prearranged hand positions, material objects, or symbols.

The purpose is to open your dharma or True Universal You so you can move forward to your highest good. You need to uncover your dharma and eliminate the negative energies that may have accumulated in your body to live your life to the fullest. Once your body, mind, and spirit are aligned, you can achieve your full potential. Remember, *you are the captain of your soul and the skipper of your fate.*

The human body is 73 to 90 percent water wherein the molecules received are attached to vibrations. Water molecules change their shape depending on the vibrations in your body. Your thoughts affect the vibrations while the water in your body readily resonates to respond to any type of vibrations.

Imagine these molecules within your body, mind, and spirit surrounded and filled with harmony and unconditional love. They can help you focus on self-healing for you to harmonize and balance your energy chakras.

Advanced Reiki doesn't only serve as a vessel wherein your universal vibrations of harmony and love flow, but it also assists you in resonating with the actual universal energy through proper techniques. Once you've learned to rely on your universal wisdom, it's easy to achieve a higher quality of life while helping improve the lives of others.

Usui Reiki energy flows through where it's needed and once the molecules have already received the amount of energy they can keep, it stops from flowing. Therefore, this energy healing technique won't cause harm to recipients. You have the free will to accept all levels of Reiki you can complete without harming yourself.

However, the universal energy won't flow if your higher self doesn't want universal harmony and love to flow through you. In other words, you cannot force Reiki on yourself or in any situation. As you practice Usui Reiki to advance your self-healing ability, your awareness also expands and the universal life force energy flows more purely without any complications.

You may fix your computer, car, or other appliances at home, but you can't fix people and other life forms. Instead, you need to simply know that Usui Reiki energy increases well-being when necessary. All you have to do is allow the universal energy to flow through you without any blockages in your mind, body, and spirit. When the emotional or the analytical mind is involved in the energy flow, inharmonious vibrations are produced.

Other terms to describe Usui Reiki include a wave of love, Reiki energy, and Reiki light. Light, life, and love are all forms of energy that are essential in a happy and healthy life. Simply put, Reiki energy is the unconditional love and light that you need to add glow to your life.

If you want to develop more powerful self-healing ability, more symbols, and miraculous experiences, the best way is to look deep within yourself. When you allow Reiki light to shine through your body without any complicated symbols or rituals, it can make a huge difference in your self-healing experience. In turn, the healing experience can help you measure your spirituality.

You can advance your self-healing ability through the following exercises:

- Trust in the universal wisdom.

- Practice the basic techniques for First Level Reiki.

- Feel your universal rhythm as well as your life rhythm.

- Allow universal harmony and love to flow through you, particularly in the areas where it is purely needed.

- Transcend training wheels including material objects, music, and symbols.

1. Practice meditations and exercises that help you know your dharma or true self.

2. Know in your heart that true knowledge must prevail instead of emotions.

To know more symbols, imagine the clock. It's a symbol that measures time and not as time itself or something that can change or create time. You might not be able to master the spiritual practice of Mikao Usui, but you solely have control over yourself, especially your mind and body. You have the power to control your mind and whatever happens in it. Therefore, the results from Usui Reiki sessions depend on your spirituality and belief that this energy healing will work.

How to Learn and Apply Advanced Reiki

Generally, there's no protocol set in stone when it comes to practicing Reiki. As long as you're ready to open yourself to the universe, you're going to create outcomes that you exactly need. There are workshops offered by Reiki masters to students who want to develop self-healing abilities, but you can also learn it yourself.

Master Attunements and advanced Reiki help strengthen an individual's connection to healing energy while boosting the benefits it can give. However, this healing technique is very simple that people from any background or age brackets can easily learn this method. During the attunement, the healing energy is transferred to the recipient from the practitioner and that's all you need to master.

If you want to connect in a deeper way with Reiki energy and help others experience the benefits, you can learn how to perform advanced Reiki. The practitioner will use the master symbols to help you transfer Empowerment Attunements and offer Healing Attunements for you to awaken other's Reiki energy.

Here's a sample of how an advanced Reiki training works:

1. During the first session, you start with meditation using Reiki symbols and hand positions. Then you will receive an attunement from the practitioner. You will also practice exercises with the practitioner as the energy increases through the master symbol. With an

increased Reiki energy, you can scan auras while sending Reiki across time and space.

2. The second session begins with the attunement, and then you will learn the practices for aura cleansing, accessing the Rainbow Bridge's power, and clearing energy. You need to familiarize yourself with the techniques and symbols so that you can effectively transmit Reiki energy throughout your body, mind, and spirit.

3. In the third session, this is where the practitioner builds a foundation with moving meditation and breath work practices. You will also learn the Tibetan Reiki symbols while receiving attunement from the Reiki practitioner. This session also involves using crystals to help you practice creating crystal grids for you to increase Reiki energy.

4. The fourth session is all about Reiki transmission energetics and empowerment attunement techniques. You will learn how to gain skill in providing attunements while integrating the techniques and symbols. Using Reiki mainly depends on attunements

so you really need to master this skill to access life force energy.

Whether you're dealing with chronic back pain or looking for some stress relief, Reiki sessions can help you achieve relaxation and pain reduction. This spiritual healing practice improves your body's healing ability by transmitting and increasing universal life energy to balance and harmonize your body, mind, and soul.

What Will You Experience During a Reiki Session?

Every Reiki session is different because there's no exact rule on how to perform it or how long it should be performed. Moreover, there's no typical environment or setting to do this healing treatment. You can choose a quiet room or any place where you feel relaxed and comfortable. Reiki can actually be done anytime and anywhere you'd like.

Some people can make Reiki appointments at a spa outlet or any place that offers this service. For first-timers, it could be a strange experience especially if you don't have any prior knowledge of what this relaxation and healing technique is all about. Usually, Reiki practitioners perform Reiki for an hour with different hand positions and some smoke from sage or other dried herbs that induce relaxation.

After blowing the smoke, your body may feel warm while there's a tingling sensation in your hands and arms. Some even experience a mysterious pressure on their chest while their legs vibrate uncontrollably. More often than not, your first experience with Reiki may be unexpected and a bit scary. But once you get the hang of it, you will eventually feel more relaxed and calm.

If you feel scared and anxious, the practitioner will explain to you why these sensations are occurring. The tensions are primarily caused by energy blockages that are being released, a clear sign that Reiki is working. It means that your body is returning to a natural state, hence the almost orgasmic energy which some people describe as a crazy feeling.

If you're curious about what's happening to the body during a Reiki session, there are a few important things you need to know.

Unlike chiropractic, acupuncture, and other alternative medicines, Reiki is not regulated. The results are often due to varied manifestations and proliferation of the practice. It is mainly influenced by historical lineages and traditions other than the background of the Reiki practitioner.

Instead of using Reiki in place of conventional treatments, it's more effective when used together in treating pain and other chronic symptoms. However, before using this with conventional treatment, it's important to clarify what it precisely is for. Avoid self-proclaimed practitioners that use blended spiritual practices and call them "reiki". Make sure that the practitioner you are going to work with only works toward single, focused practice.

The overall experience can be described as a shamanic practice or energy medicine where the Reiki master transmits the energy and clears obstructions. If it's practiced with less intervention and more on reestablishing the energy in the recipient, there will be stronger healing results. However, the practitioner will only assist you in harnessing the energy by releasing stress and relaxing the mind, body, and spirit.

Your body will move or shake during a Reiki session due to the fluctuations of life force energy or energy shift. If you're looking for a scientific explanation for this, there's simply no answer. On the other hand, the mind will deal with the rituals and symbols of medicine while the practitioner activates the brain's neurotransmitters and specific regions that produce these neurotransmitters.

What you can expect from a Reiki session is reduced stress, fatigue, and pain rather than curing your medical condition such as cancer. In addition, the physical sensations that you experience during the treatment is because your body is releasing energy.

Visually, the universe shows the recipient the universal energy that is already present in the body but most people are not aware of this. As mentioned in the previous chapters, different vibrations are represented by different colors. Even so, the colors have no power just like the symbols used in performing the healing session. The colors demonstrate the pieces of life force energy flowing through the body called Usui Reiki.

It's not recommended to combine hand positions with flames. Rather, it's better to resonate with the reality of life force energy and realize where it's taking you.

You can compare mastering advanced Reiki with sculpting. Here's an ideal way to do Reiki through carving:

- Start with a specific form or block that represents your body, mind, and spirit.

- Take away some pieces from that form that you think is not needed. It could be a negative belief or any complicated emotions.

- Continue removing the parts that keep you from discovering your inner beauty.

- Once you've completely eliminated all the negative including worry and anger, self-healing begins so you can reveal your dharma or True Universal Self.

- Take time to sand and polish the form for you to achieve the outcome that you want. No matter what shape or form you have created, see it as a beautiful creation because it uniquely represents you.

The brain has different sects wherein memory is stored while the heart is where true knowledge is found. This is the main reason why learning advanced Reiki healing is essential in understanding the different vibrations you will experience throughout the session. The techniques and exercises are all important in creating the exact outcome you need.

Harmony and balance make this spiritual practice more meaningful and beautiful. Imagine the entire universe in perfect harmony, there will surely be world peace. When you acknowledge inharmonious and harmonious vibrations while trusting in universal wisdom, the ground where you are standing seems much different than it was before.

When life throws you a lemon, you should learn to be flexible and move in the rhythm of harmony and love so you can live your life to the fullest. When there is a storm, learn how to dance in the rain. If you're dealing with challenges, it's always important to be optimistic and hopeful. By honoring the universal energy and recognizing it within you, no amount of difficulty can make you feel powerless.

Undergoing a Reiki session will introduce you to new things that you didn't know exist in you. In case you're still unaware, there are secrets in your existence that you need to discover for you to know the real you. So don't be afraid to get to know yourself more through Reiki healing. You will surely enjoy uncovering your inner truths while strengthening your energy so you can live happier and healthier.

From Whom Should You Receive Advanced Reiki?

For you to make sure that you're going to have a result-driven experience, you should find a certified Reiki practitioner with knowledge in this healing practice. You can choose a professional Reiki master or a friend who knows how to properly conduct a Reiki session. The important thing is that you feel comfortable with the person you want to receive Reiki from.

The level of experience of your friend might not be the same as the experience of a professional practitioner, but the comfort it may give you is surely unmatched. Plus, receiving Reiki treatment from your friend is a good bonding experience. However, make sure that your friend clearly understands the process and can walk you through each step of the session for you to achieve the best experience.

The actual experience during a Reiki therapy is personal and very subjective. Meaning, your experience will never be the same as with other recipients' experiences. Therefore, you really need to choose a practitioner who knows what they're doing so that you will get the level of relaxation and calmness you need.

A trustworthy Reiki practitioner knows the ideal setting to conduct a session. Usually, a quiet space is the best place to receive Reiki as long as no disturbance or noise can interrupt the session. If you don't have a quiet place, don't worry because most practitioners offer a dedicated setting where recipients can relax while receiving Reiki.

If practitioners make house calls, they can create that space with some soft music to mask ambient noises. However, if you like silence, just tell your practitioner so that a more ideal and comfortable setting will be created for you. If you're undergoing a Reiki session in a healthcare setting such as a nursing home, hospice, or hospital, you will be given a short session which only takes up to 20 minutes to finish. On the other hand, some private practitioners offer 90-minutes Reiki sessions.

Practitioners with healthcare training may conduct health interviews or provide intake forms for you to focus on what you exactly need such as pain reduction or stress relief. But since this healing therapy is conducted as folk practice, many practitioners avoid any types of intake that are common in the healthcare industry. Instead, you will be given a form of consent which you need to sign before the session.

More often than not, practitioners explain the whole process to the recipient to give them an idea of what to expect. If you want to address specific needs, better let your practitioner know. Have open communication with your practitioner so that there will be no problem during the session, especially if you have certain health issues. For instance, your body may have specific parts that are highly sensitive for hands-on therapy.

Each Reiki session consists of hand positions and symbols that increase the life force energy in the body. A complete session is given to a fully-clothed patient sitting in a chair or lying comfortably on a table. Most commonly, it's given through a non-invasive touch while the hands of the practitioner are held on specific parts of the head, front torso, and lower back.

The hand positions should be light and not intrusive or giving too much pressure on the body. Other hand positions can be placed on your limbs for you to soothe injuries and other pain points. If necessary, the practitioner will hold their hands off the body to heal a burn or an open wound.

Your experience with your Reiki practitioner should be refreshing and relaxing. Some recipients even fall asleep due to the very relaxing experience during the session. It's like having a massage that soothes every muscle and joint that is aching. Again, experiences are subjective and may depend on the recipient's condition.

The hands of practitioners doing a Reiki are often warm, but there are times that they feel cool. Some recipients also experience subtle pulsations throughout their bodies while the hands of the practitioner are placed on areas with cascading vibrations.

Is there any difference between the pioneer Reiki teachers and the practitioners of today? When Reiki became known from Japan to different parts of the world, practitioners have slightly modified the original technique that Usui Sensei developed. However, no one ever claims to be more effective or better than the others.

There's no secret in performing a Reiki session, but rather the process can be described as astonishing, amazing, or humbling. When you allow the universal energy to flow through you, it simply makes you feel natural and calm. If you're dealing with a physical challenge that the health experts say can no longer be cured, Reiki will help you experience happiness by reducing stress and tension in your body.

Now, how long should you receive Reiki?

Practitioners may recommend a series of Reiki sessions for you to heal you from depression, anxiety, and pain that are causing you more distress aside from the physical challenges you are having. The traditional recommendation is four sessions to have enough time to assess your condition and what benefits you're getting.

It's important to talk to your practitioner about the expectations you have and how you want to be treated. For instance, describe what kind of setting you want to do Reiki as well as the ideal schedule that suits your needs. In case of a severe medical problem, Reiki practitioners may conduct four sessions for four days for you to address the problems. However, you may get a new practitioner if you feel you're not comfortable with the previous one.

You can't visually see the atoms in your body, mind, and spirit. Similarly, you can't know the exact source of your symptoms that are occurring. The good news is that you don't need to know or see them. Reiki healing is administered through universal wisdom which knows how and where to flow through so that your symptoms will be healed.

Chapter 8 - Energy Medicine: The Future of Alternative Therapy

What is Energy Medicine?

Energy medicine refers to various practices that were derived from complementary medical theories. The term was first used in the 80s when the International Society for the Study of Subtle Engines and Energy Medicine was also founded.

This type of treatment comes in different forms, but they mainly fall into the main categories namely: putative and veritable.

Veritable energy medicine refers to the specific energetic forms including magnetic or light therapy which are measurable. On the other hand, putative energy medicine can't be measured.

Western medicine involves different forms of energy. Sound waves help visualize certain areas in the body using sonograms. If you're suffering from disorders like Seasonal Affective Disorder, light therapy can be used to improve your mood during months when sunlight is limited. Other forms of energy medicine that are veritable include an electromagnetic pulse of static magnet therapy.

Reiki therapy falls under the form of energy medicine that is putative. This works with the help of energy fields that every individual has. A blocked or disturbed energy field can lead to certain diseases and ailments. Therefore, the practitioner needs to restore harmony and balance within the energy field.

Up to date, alternative and putative medical interventions are significantly increasing. They are focused on creating well-balanced energy fields or Ki in the body of patients. The most common therapies that are now gaining even more popularity around the world include emotional freedom therapy, qi gong, distance healing, therapeutic massage, acupuncture, homeopathy, and Reiki therapy. These therapies are developed to help restore the body's balance by clearing blockages in the energy fields.

If you consider these therapies, you will realize why the other form of energy medicine is categorized as putative. That is because there's simply no way to measure how much or how you are using energy through these therapies unlike veritable forms of energy medicine. Also, there's a difference between praying for a sick person and using electromagnetic pulses to cure a person.

You might be asking how many prayers you need to heal, or how long or often should you pray. Again, there are no measurable answers you can get to such questions. This is also what practitioners will surely tell you about putative therapies.

With the numerous techniques used in energy medicine, it's not easy to distinguish facts from fiction when determining the efficacy of a specific method. In addition, there are different standards you can apply for you to test the effectiveness of such techniques. Some therapies like homeopathy may interact with other medications and medical conditions.

If you're drained, energy medicine can bring you vitality, joy when you're depressed, and health when you're sick. It also awakens your life force energy for you to become happy, enthusiastic, and resilient. When your body, mind, and soul are balanced, your energies will flow freely and regulate your hormones. As a result, you feel much better and think more clearly.

As a self-healing and development way to better health and growth, energy medicine empowers people to adapt to new health challenges and thrive within a healthy environment focused on balancing energy fields. To maintain your vitality, here are some tips to help your body manage its energies:

- Have enough space to move around to avoid being inactive. If you live a sedentary lifestyle, your energies will be plugged with toxins. Blocked life force energy can lead to prolonged stress and interference from negative energies.

- Move in harmony with physical functions and structures that the universal energy support and invigorate. Keep in mind that flow follows purpose.

- Touch on all levels including the micro-level which is represented by DNA and the macro level which relates to the left brain controlling the body's right side and vice versa.

- Maintain balance with all the energies in your body. With prolonged stress and other health issues, the universal energy may lose its natural balance. Therefore, you need to keep your energy fields perfectly balanced.

- Stay healthy to prevent disturbances from affecting your energies.

Energy medicine involves certain techniques from historical traditions including kinesiology, yoga, and Reiki. It acknowledges energy as an essential moving force to determine things like happiness and health. Harmony, balance, and flow can be achieved through non-invasive methods to restore and maintain healthy energy systems.

Is Energy Medicine the Future of Health and Healing?

Once you learn how to enter the subtle energies within your body, you can easily connect to your eternal essence as well as spiritual callings. There's no particular religious affiliation, allegiance, or belief system that you need to use in energy medicine. All you need is to believe that it's going to work for you to get results.

Anyone can do energy medicine as long as they understand the fundamentals of this natural healing method. It's your birthright to work with your life force energy to live a satisfying life. Below is a list of people who can perform energy medicine:

- Ordinary people without any experience or knowledge of energy healing.

- People who want to develop their self-healing ability and use life force energy for vitality and health.

- Anyone who likes to master techniques that can help them heal others, especially friends and family.

- Everyone who plans to build a career or long-term practice in energy medicine.

- Healthcare experts who want to offer alternative healing to patients with depression, chronic pain, and anxiety.

- Doctors, nurses, acupuncturists, and massage therapists who want to enhance and level up their skills.

Some of the most common hands-on techniques of energy medicine are to tap, massage, pinch, twist, or connect specific energies in your body. You can trace or swirl your hands over your skin through energy pathways to heal acupoints. In addition, you can perform some postures or exercises for you to create specific effects that help balance your mind, body, and spirit.

Now, is energy medicine really the future of healing?

Many people are saying that energy medicine is the *"medicine of the future"*. While it empowers people today by helping them adapt to health challenges, energy medicine is still a work in progress for scientists in proving its benefits.

But let's focus on why people are calling it the future of medicine.

When you acknowledge the invisible energies in your body, the cells become happy, the systems or organs are in harmony, and the heart starts to release positive emotions. It's not hard to understand why practitioners and even healthcare workers are now realizing the advantages of energy medicine in healing people.

According to health practitioners, the medical field is soon to collapse due to the ugly politics happening behind it. However, they believe that the Higher Power has a plan for all of us. It's a good practice to have faith in Him and that His healing powers will save us all. To achieve true healing, it's important to believe that God has given us an innate gift – and that self-healing.

With the increasing awareness of people with regards to the efficacy of energy medicine, healthcare practitioners feel that it's going to become more mainstream. They are even excited that this alternative medicine could become a go-to healing method and may take over big pharmaceuticals.

Energy medicine is simply bringing people back to acknowledge their innate wisdom. The human body is an inner healer, you just need to recognize its amazing ability to improve your health and provide an ideal environment where your energies can thrive.

By creating a space for your body to recover and heal, energy medicine calms the mind and helps the spirit to prosper. It fixes the body by removing toxins and clearing out blockages in the pathways. When you connect with your inner life force and accept the real you, it's possible to prevent illnesses and negative emotions that impact the quality of your life.

Scientists are even getting closer to solid evidence that there's more than surgery and medicine to heal people. Illnesses are often caused by emotional or mental factors, which is why more studies are being conducted to arrive at the best conclusion.

Another reason for the growing popularity of energy medicine is the continuing shortage of medical doctors in the field. Therefore, holistic integrative therapies are becoming more essential in treating illnesses. This important modality can help reduce the need for drug treatment, particularly Western medicine.

Indeed, the future is bright for energy medicine as various parts of the world are recognizing it in healing people from certain health problems. More and more people are becoming aware of the real essence of energy in achieving optimum health.

Therapeutic touch, healing touch, or whatever names you call Reiki therapy, it has become widely known as an energy medicine technique that helps improve symptoms of high blood pressure, heart conditions, and other common illnesses.

Hospitals that Offer Energy Medicine

The American Hospital Association recorded more than 800 hospitals that offered Reiki healing as part of their hospital services in 2007 across America. These clinics and hospitals accept the cost-effective advantage that Reiki offers in improving patient care.

In some interviews with healthcare professionals, they say that Reiki sessions help patients recover faster from their medical conditions while reducing painful symptoms. This energy healing therapy also reduces the side effects of certain medications and boosts the mental attitude of patients.

Some nurses include Reiki in their regular nursing routines as per the request of patients. Through word-of-mouth, more patients as well as hospital staff have accepted the treatment to speed up the recovery process. They conduct the sessions in recovery and operating rooms to increase the efficacy of the therapeutic touch.

Some nurses do Reiki on patients with cancer and bone marrow transplants at the Memorial Sloane Kettering Hospital. For the record, there were 26 nurses and 6 doctors in the hospital who practice Reiki as part of patient care services.

So, how interested is America in complementary patient care?

People in the United States are becoming more interested in complementary healthcare practices such as Reiki therapy. According to a study which was headed by Dr. David Eisenberg at the Beth Israel Hospital in Boston, one out of three Americans uses energy healing. The study shows there were more than 14 billion dollars spent on alternative medicine in 1990.

Another survey revealed that 161,000 children and 1.2 million adults in America received Reiki sessions in 2006. The wider acceptance of energy healing is clearly establishing ground in the medical field. With more hospitals incorporating Reiki therapy in their patient services, there's no surprise if the number of

Reiki-trained doctors and nurses continues to increase.

In fact, in the mid-1990s, Reiki has already been used in operating rooms to help patients reduce surgical pains and other physical symptoms. Since then, the recognition of energy medicine has grown over the years. Currently, it's listed in the medical publication as part of the nursing practice scope and standards. You can check out the Center for Reiki Research website to see the complete list of hospitals that currently offer Reiki therapy and other energy healing techniques.

There are certain reasons why hospitals and other healthcare institutions are interested in offering Reiki to patients. For instance, many hospitals are currently undergoing improvements in their services and experiencing major changes in patient care programs to cut costs.

Under the traditional medical model, expensive technology and medication practices pose an unsolvable problem. The solution is to offer complimentary modalities such as Reiki for you to implement cost-effective methods. Obviously, Reiki healing doesn't need any technology for you to achieve results. Plus, the training services of practitioners are free. Therefore, energy medicine is a perfect way to achieve the cost-cutting goals of hospitals.

Cardiothoracic surgeon Mehmet Oz of the Columbia Presbyterian Medical Center worked with Reiki Master Julie Motz to help balance the energies of patients during operations. They also use other energy medicine techniques for you to reduce pain during heart transplants and open-heart surgery.

According to Motz, all heart patients that were treated with Reiki did not experience postoperative depression, organ rejection, leg weakness, and postoperative pain. The subtle energy medicine techniques used in operating rooms led to positive thoughts and feelings among the patients, hence increasing the trust gained from medical practitioners as well as patients.

Oncologist David Guillon of Marin General Hospital stated that he feels the need to exhaust all efforts for you to help their patients. While they are providing modern health care methods, energy healing remains an essential part of the recovery of patients. Therefore, he endorses the potential benefits of Reiki therapy to aid people in using their energies to overcome health challenges.

Portsmouth Regional Hospital in New Hampshire is another health facility where Reiki is offered. A registered nurse and Reiki master Patricia Alandydy works as the Assistant Director of Surgical Services in the hospital. She was the one who initiated that the hospital should offer Reiki services to patients under her department.

The surgical services department is a large section in the hospital which covers the post-surgery floor, Ambulatory Care Unit, Post-anesthesia Care Unit, Central Supply, and the operating rooms. When they conduct telephone interviews with patients, Dr.

Alandydy makes sure that the services offered include Reiki.

If the patient requests energy healing treatment, it is automatically included in their admission during their surgery and then a 20-minute session before they are brought to the surgery room. Some sessions are also conducted in operating rooms to help patients relax and get ready for the surgery procedure.

Medical practitioners say that giving Reiki to patients is a rewarding experience. It's impressive how patients and other people embrace the potential of energy healing in pain reduction and fast recoveries. This goes to show that more people are open-minded to complementary modalities despite not seeing these so-called energies.

Top Schools That Offer Energy Medicine Courses

The National Center for Complementary and Alternative Medicine considers energy healing a variety of alternative medicine. There are graduate programs offered in different colleges for those who want to earn applicable credentials for you to practice energy medicine such as Reiki treatment.

If you want to get a formal education on energy healing, here are some pointers to consider when choosing a school for energy medicine:

- The school should be accredited for energy medicine graduate programs. There are specific requirements the school needs to meet before they can officially offer such courses.

- Determine your ultimate career goal. Some alternative medicine techniques are taught beyond mainstream medical training while other forms are taught according to traditional medical education.

- Complementary and alternative medicine programs accept students with an undergraduate degree related to pre-medicine and nursing.

Now, what are the programs you can choose from to get your certificate in energy medicine?

Certified Healing Touch Practitioner Program is a voluntary certification you can earn to become a *Certified Healing Touch Practitioner*. Typically, CHTPs have 5 certification levels. Once you earn all 5 levels, you can become an energy medicine instructor.

Master's Degree in Integrative Medicine is available for nurses, researchers, healthcare providers, and physicians who want to complete an integrative medicine education. Some master's degree courses offer practicum, research, and publication opportunities.

Master of Science in Nursing, Holistic Nursing is a program where nurses are trained to practice clinical or advanced nursing specializations. This curriculum includes laboratory and community practicum requirements. Some colleges teach different modalities for energy medicine or offer specialized programs for energy medicine.

The following are some of the top schools that offer related programs and courses in fields of integrative and complementary medicine:

- Mount Wachusett Community College in Gardner Maryland offers certificate and Associate's degree for two years.

- University of East-West Medicine in Sunnyvale, California offers Master's degree for 4 years.

- American College of Healthcare Sciences in Portland, Oregon offers a Master's Certificate degree for 4 years. However, this is for distance learning program only.

- National University of Health Sciences in Lombard, Illinois offers Doctorate degree for 4 years.

- Maryland University of Integrative Health in Laurel, Maryland offers a Master's degree for 4 years.

- Drexel University in Philadelphia, Pennsylvania offers a Certificate degree for 4 years.

When choosing an energy medicine program, it's important to verify the accreditation level of the school or college you plan to enroll. Also, check the prerequisites of the course or program for you to ensure the outcomes and coursework match your career goals. There are various programs and degrees offered to suit the types of job titles you want to apply once you earned your energy medicine degree or certificate.

What is the curriculum for energy medicine courses?

- *Energy Medicine Practitioner, Advanced Diploma Program.* This holistic energy medicine curriculum is focused on complementary and alternative medicine. It covers Human Energy Field Testing such as screening devices to accurately and completely test body systems for wellness evaluation.

- o The only requirement you need to enroll in this curriculum is your GED or high school diploma. The average duration is between 9 to 18 months with 44 total credit hours. The course outline includes kinesiology, reflexology, digestive wellness, chemistry and nutrition, pathology, and natural health to name a few.

- *Energy Medicine Consultant.* This curriculum is for students who want to apply bio-energetic methods to wellness. It consists of e-book courses to aid in distance learning. You only need a GED or high school diploma to enroll in this program for 5 to 6 months average duration.

  - o The course outline includes chemistry basics, anatomy and physiology, micro-circulation enhancement, Bach flower remedies, and PEMF therapy to name a few. The total credit for this program is 19 hours.

- *Certified Homeopathic Consultant.* This certificate program teaches students to provide homeopathic guidance to patients. It's a 9-course curriculum that only requires GED or high school diploma to enroll. It takes 3 to 6 months for you to complete the course and get your certificate.

    o The course outline includes dietary wellness for life, homeopathy, natural health methods, cell salts, homeopathic remedies, and business practice for natural health to name a few. The total credit for this curriculum is 17 hours only.

Some hospitals and healthcare facilities are offering college tuition, free housing, and signing bonuses for you to retain medical workers. If you're currently working as a nurse and you want to become a professional Reiki healer or energy healer, you can check with your employer if they're offering these perks. More nursing graduates with a background in energy medicine are needed now than ever.

Chapter 9 - Reiki Side Effects

Are There Side Effects of Reiki Healing

Side effects are phenomena or occurrences that are not pleasant. For instance, conventional treatments and medicinal drugs may have certain side effects such as diarrhea, nausea, and kidney damage. However, some side effects are unavoidable and are part of the treatments.

So, are there any side effects when you use Reiki treatment?

As a non-invasive and natural healing technique, Reiki may still have some side effects on recipients. While there are proven benefits of using energy healing, there are also a few negative affects you need to consider before trying it.

However, you may call them pleasant side effects because they actually rejuvenate the body despite the unpleasant physical symptoms that are experienced. In addition, these side effects are not only physical but can also be emotional and mental.

After the attunement, Reiki practitioners periodically experience specific side effects in their lifetime. Nevertheless, they are experienced more intensely after the session. The following are the most common side effects that you may experience from Reiki healing:

- Less energy.

- Fatigue and grogginess.

- Light-headedness.

- Stomach upset and other abdominal disturbances.

- Fever.

- Sore throat and cold.

- Pain in the body, specifically in the head and heart.

- The emergence of old emotional-mental patterns that are unhealthy.

- Changes in relationships, personal life, career, and more.

Every recipient may experience different side effects because healing is not the same for everyone. You experience certain symptoms that others did not get to experience because what happens to you is what's necessary to help you heal from your unique condition.

To explain it further, the cells in your body carry particular imprints of your experiences that may span several lifetimes. Most of these imprints tend to be self-sabotaging, karmic, and plainly negative. You may not be aware of this, but you are likely to carry a load of negative energies before experiencing the benefits of Reiki healing.

The attunement helps you see the light and break away from the dark world that succumbed to you for some time. Once the Reiki light enters your body, the negative cells automatically leave your entire being. This is when the healing happens, while the side effects slowly disappear.

However, the process of healing may take a long time before it is completed as there are stages you need to overcome. Every time you heal, a layer of the negative aura is released while experiencing the side effects. There's a break in between these healing stages to help the body advance to the next layer.

Each layer that is released may give different side effects, so be prepared for this. Your body will gradually flush out all the toxins in your cells for you to pave the way for a stronger immune system, higher quality of life, and greater wellness.

Therefore, there's really no need to worry about the aftereffects of Reiki therapy because they are part of the healing process. Instead, welcome whatever is happening on the surface to make sure your body, mind, and spirit experience is properly cleansed and healed.

For you to understand what Reiki does to your body during a session, here are some detailed accounts of the potential side effects of energy healing:

- You may feel some discomfort during Reiki. To perform the treatment, you will be asked to lay down on the table inside a dim room. As the Reiki master stands over your body, you should not make any unnecessary movements. There may be mellow music played to help you calm down during the session. While holding still, it can make you feel uncomfortable which may cause panic and anxiety attacks.

- Reduced oxygen level in the blood. One of the negative placebo effects of Reiki treatment is low levels of oxygen in the blood. This was reported in a clinical trial conducted in 2013 with children who underwent dental procedures.

- Increased fatigue and weakness. While most recipients feel calm and relaxed after the treatment, some feel tired and weak. According to Reiki practitioners, this is due to the healing effects in the body. Increased fatigue and weakness may come with headaches, nausea, and stomach pain.

Alternative medicine such as Reiki is developed to increase the self-healing ability of the body so that maladies will be cured with less physical symptoms. However, the detoxifying cleanse that comes with the healing process may give some unpleasant side effects.

Ideally, the body will work harder for you to heal from certain health conditions. While accomplishing true healing, it's inevitable to experience some cleansing aftereffects. Therefore, these side effects that Reiki may have aren't really bad at all. Not to worry, these effects will only last a short time; some even disappear in one day after the treatment.

Awkward Symptoms of Reiki Attunement

Some websites claim Reiki therapy doesn't have any potential risks since it's a non-intrusive healing technique. More often than not, the effects highlighted for energy healing are relaxation and calmness. So, are there symptoms the body may experience when doing Reiki attunements?

During attunements, recipients will experience a cleansing or detoxifying effects. Therefore, it's important to understand the cautions before undergoing any alternative medicine treatments. Some people endure the aftereffects for up to 3 weeks while others have a shorter duration.

If you have serious health problems, you need to consult your doctor before getting an energy healing treatment. Attunements can worsen the current symptoms you have as your body may respond differently to the treatment. The best way to get the desired result is to talk to your practitioner and be open to the potential symptoms you will experience after the treatment.

The attunement opens your chakras to allow the universal energy to heal your body. By releasing all the toxins in your body, detoxification can be an unpleasant experience just like when you're having withdrawal symptoms from caffeine or other unhealthy foods.

Another potential risk of energy medicine is that you may develop mental dependence on your healer despite the insufficient evidence that it actually works. There are websites that say energy healing is a scam and is perpetrated by fraudsters. However, there are studies to bust these negative claims and it's up to you whether to believe them or not.

The following are potential risks of Reiki attunement:

- The physical symptoms that recipients may experience during attunements include cold or warm hands and feet, tingling sensations, and buzzing of specific body parts.

  Others also experience chest pain, headaches, cranial pressure, runny nose, blurred vision, diarrhea, and limb stiffness. It's important to know that the higher the toxicity level the body contains, the more physical symptoms will be experienced.

- The emotional symptoms of Reiki attunements include sadness, anger outbursts, fear, frustration, and crying for no reason. These intense emotions are common when you undergo attunements because it's part of the healing process – letting go of negative energies that bring you down.

Traumas and other deep emotions that are suppressed will be aggravated during attunements before they completely disappear. For you to clear unsettled emotions, they need to pass through your body. While they reemerge, you will experience such emotions including depression, anger, fear, and sadness.

However, it's normal to feel these emotions after the attunement. So there's no need to panic or be harsh on yourself because it's actually helping you heal from past traumas. Your practitioner will guarantee that emotional detoxification after Reiki attunements is temporary.

- In terms of energetical symptoms, you may experience high vibrations after a Reiki attunement. Your body releases deeply buried negative energies for you to balance your mind, body, and spirit. Once it's been completed, you are likely to experience a stronger vibe in your body.

  When you're at a higher vibration, you will notice people behaving like an energy vampire sucking up your energy. The good thing is that they can't easily drain your energy because you're energized by Reiki. Also, you no longer want to get involved in other people's dramas.

  Instead, you start to set boundaries for you to keep toxic people from affecting your life negatively. It's important to surround yourself with friends who uplift you and help you become a better person.

However, when you're at a higher vibration, you may attract those with low vibrations like a flame attracting the moth.

Your most vulnerable moment is when you sleep. Therefore, make sure to condition your mind before going to bed that you will be joined by spiritual masters and angels while you're asleep.

- Some changes in your spiritual beliefs may also be experienced after the attunement. However, receiving and giving Reiki isn't a religion, but rather a mere spiritual experience. There's no need to adopt some beliefs for you to practice this energy healing technique.

  However, you may create some new spiritual beliefs after the session. For instance, you may believe that you are basically your own ego, something you identify yourself with as the person that you really are.

- There might also be some radical shifts you will experience in your life due to the vibrational changes in your body. For instance, you might suddenly shift your career path or decide to start your own business. Some even choose to be a Reiki healer as their life purpose.

  Whatever it is that your soul is searching for, be passionate about achieving your goals. The earth will make a way to help you find your true calling while guiding you in your relationships with living things, including animals and plants.

If it's your first time getting a Reiki treatment, it's good to ask your healer regarding the potential symptoms you might experience after the attunement. Also, let him know if you have a serious health condition to avoid putting your life at risk in case the side effects of Reiki aggravate your existing condition.

As mentioned earlier, the aftereffects of Reiki attunements are normal and can never be avoided. Mental purification, for instance, needs the mind to release energy-sucking thoughts, toxins, and emotions. During the cleansing process, some unhealthy habits may reappear such as cravings for sugary foods and drinking alcohol.

You need to resist going back to these old habits as they will only create worse side effects after a Reiki treatment. Pessimistic thoughts also lead to a mental burden that can make you feel heavy and reluctant in opening up yourself to positive energies.

With regular Reiki treatments or daily practice of this healing technique, you can discover some spiritual insights within yourself. Remember, what you see in other people reflects your own image. If you're noticing some patterns of negative energies in other people, it's your chance to identify your own demons so you can free yourself from similar patterns of negativity.

Now, is there any way to reduce the side effects of Reiki attunements?

Meditation is your number one friend during such challenging times. You need to stay optimistic when dealing with negative energies. But more importantly, you should develop a healthy lifestyle for you to feel your best. Here are some effective ways to reduce the side effects of Reiki:

- Sleep early and see to it that you are getting enough sleep everyday. To help your mind relax during the attunement, a healthy sleeping habit can help a lot.

- Stop smoking or drinking alcohol, especially at night. It will disturb your energy and cause mood swings and headaches.

- Avoid eating animal-based proteins and other high-protein foods to aid the body during the healing process.

- Eat a well-balanced diet with lots of vegetables and fruits for you to boost your immune system and keep infections and other health problems at bay.

- Stop drinking caffeinated drinks such as coffee, soft drinks, some teas, energy drinks, and cocoa. Do this at least one week prior to your Reiki treatment because caffeine can make your mind overactive.

But wait, not all side effects of Reiki attunements are negative. Below are the beneficial aftereffects of doing a Reiki:

- During the first level of Reiki attunement, the effects include third eye-opening, new mental powers, increased intuition, and positive changes in eating habits. Basically, level one opens up the mind chakra, expands the energy center, and introduces the recipient to a different flow of energy.

- The aftereffects of the second level of Reiki attunement include increased feelings of empathy and compassion, enhanced connection to other living things, sudden mood swings, and varying levels of energy. This level opens up the heart chakra and makes the recipient more aware of his emotions and feelings that are hidden or unrecognized.

- On the third level of Reiki attunement, the effects include a feeling of lightness, strengthened connection to everything, deeper understanding, higher consciousness, and the ability to see energy chakras. As the master level of Reiki attunement, this is the stage where you experience continuous energy flow.

Despite the side effects, Reiki masters say that these outcomes after the attunements are not permanent—

most of them only last for several days. Once your body is used to the new energy flow and consciousness level, you will feel rejuvenated and healed.

To help detoxify your body, even more, you can meditate, take warm baths, and do some breathing exercises to eliminate the toxins. In addition, it's also recommended to drink more water and stop eating sugary foods as they can disrupt your energy chakras. You can do yoga to maintain a healthy state of mind while enhancing the positive effects of Reiki attunements.

As you begin to learn and master this energy healing method, you will understand the inner works of your body and mind. For example, you will learn the best ways to heal from various medical issues while progressing on your spiritual path.

Day in and day out, you are guided by your life force energy. If you practice Reiki daily, you increase your connection with Reiki energy which can lead you to miracles and more beneficial effects.

The better you are able to release the negative energies in your body, the more effective the cleansing process becomes. As a result, you enjoy the freedom from any past traumas that hold you back. You are headed to a straight, well-lit path that leads to unending happiness and optimum health.

When you believe that Reiki is going to work before even starting the treatment, you will see better outcomes right after. More importantly, you should do this in a comfortable environment where you are free to be yourself without any reservations.

Tips to Protect Yourself When Doing Reiki

Many recipients wonder what happens during a Reiki session. They are clueless about what to expect or experience from this type of energy healing method. Therefore, people are often unwilling to undergo this treatment because they're afraid of what might happen. Well, this is perfectly understandable.

First of all, there are general safety guidelines that you need to consider before you try Reiki for the first time. This will help you get an idea of what to expect before, during, and after the session. Remember, fear is usually the product of a lack of understanding, education, or knowledge. With the right information on alternative therapies like Reiki, you will be confident when making decisions on whether or not to undergo such treatment.

Being involved in your healing program helps you become more responsible and active in the entire treatment. It's important that you are also participating during the treatment instead of just letting your practitioner do all the work and expect a miracle.

You need to be involved in the process so you can achieve the exact results you want. Also, you will need a protection plan to help ensure you are getting a safe treatment from a certified practitioner. The plan should include proper cleansing and balancing of your physical, mental, emotional, and spiritual health.

Usually, the aftereffects of Reiki tend to disappear in 48 hours. However, if you are experiencing some unpleasant side effects, you can do the following to help you recover and heal in a better and faster way:

- Drink at least 8 glasses of water daily for you to eliminate the toxins from the body. It also helps in stimulating better energy flow throughout the different chakras.

- Spend more time alone to refrain from absorbing the negative energies of other people.

- Make sure to take more rest time everyday to assist the physical body in opening up the energy channels.

- Pamper yourself and relax by listening to music, taking a warm bath, having a reflexology therapy, or getting a massage.

- Read some good books, go for a walk, or get a sauna bath.

- Do some cool hobbies such as gardening, swimming, and painting.

There are people that say Reiki can be dangerous if you do it with an amateur practitioner. There are different stories about energy healing that makes some people skeptical about choosing this alternative therapy. However, if you choose a reliable practitioner to help you open your chakras and allow the universal energy to flow through you, then you will get positive results.

The ideal daily protection plan mainly consists of grounding, cleansing, and protecting yourself. Before starting your day, it's important to take time to condition your body, mind, and spirit for you to avoid negative vibrations and energies in your surroundings.

One of the most common methods in grounding is the tree root. Get a chair and sit comfortably, but you can also do this while standing. Take three deep breaths while your eyes are closed. The focus and intention should be to imagine tree roots and spread them from the root chakra to the feet until they reach the earth's center. Visualize the roots scattering in every direction while they attach to the center of the earth. Know and feel that you're grounded to the energies of the earth.

To help cleanse your body, mind, and soul, you can practice the waterfall method. Get a chair and sit comfortably, but you can also do this while standing. Take three deep breaths while your eyes are closed. Imagine you are under the waterfalls. The focus and intention should be to acknowledge and feel the water as it washes and cleanses your body.

Visualize the energy blockages that are washed away as well as the low vibrating energies including toxins trapped in your body. As the energies flow through the earth's center, they will turn into higher vibrations or positive energy which you can use in case of need. You can do this several times everyday for you to make sure you don't absorb any negative energies that can make you feel uneasy and irritable.

To protect yourself, you can do the bubble of the color method. Take three deep breaths while your eyes are closed. Imagine yourself being surrounded by a bubble of color, choose any color that appeals to you. Visualize another person being surrounded by a different color to separate their energy from yours.

Feel and recognize that you're protected from low vibrating energies all the time. This will help you maintain harmony and balance in your life force energy as well as your mind, body, and spirit. Don't forget to meditate regularly so that you can focus on the good things around you instead of the negative vibrations.

Chapter 10 - How to Fix Leaking Energy and Close the Holes in Your Aura

What is a Leaking Energy

Are you experiencing a sudden drain of energy lately? Do you feel like you're in a fight or flight mode all the time? Perhaps, you are having panic or anxiety attacks that worsen your health condition. If that's the case, you may have leaking energy.

People with leaking energy may lose significant weight while suffering from burn out and break downs. This can be caused by widely opened chakras where the universal energy leaks. You may also have this weird feeling that something is leaking within your body.

Deep down your core self, you can sense the importance of sustaining and retaining your energy fields. But what do these holes in your chakras really mean?

It's good to start knowing the aura before going through the leaking energy fields in your body. The physical body comes with an "etheric double" which penetrates and extends up to 2 centimeters from the body. It serves as a template, but it also contains every organ of the body in energy form. In addition, the etheric double has chakras and meridians as well.

The universal life force energy flows throughout the body's etheric double with subtle electrical currents that invigorate the body. At the same time, it also completes the physiological processes needed to maintain energy flow in the body. This etheric double is very important for the physical body as all disorders and defects are manifested by both the body and its etheric double.

The aura of the etheric double is referred to as the etheric aura which is made up of multiple layers. The main protective layer is called the Golden Web which protects you from any harmful beings and energies around you.

Your etheric body is the bridge between your astral or emotional body and your physical body. Therefore, your etheric body including its aura can influence your psychological and physical states. For instance, if your etheric body is contaminated with toxins, you will feel sick and baffled.

Your words, actions, emotions, and thoughts influence your etheric body including your meridians, chakras, and organs. An ideal etheric body resonates at higher vibrations which allow it to create free energy flow throughout the body. Your aura should be clean, dense, strong, and smooth. However, most people's auras today are far from being smooth and clean so Reiki is essential.

More commonly, ordinary people who don't practice energy healing have uneven and congested auras with holes and cracks in their chakras. Let's say you are always in front of your computer which exposes you to radiation. This could breach your aura in the chest, solar plexus, and head.

There are different sizes of holes in your aura, they can be as tiny as a pinhole or as big as an open wound. These holes can make you more vulnerable to negative energies while leaking the positive energy in your body.

The following are the most common reasons why you have leaking energy:

- channeling

- black magic or intentional attacks

- unintentional psychic attacks such as criticism, negative thoughts

- electromagnetic fields

- environmental toxins

- missing soul fragments

- pharmacological agents

- anesthesia

- drugs and alcohol

- psychological traumas

- strong emotions such as fear, anger

Apparently, there are potential dangers if you have holes in your aura, particularly in the Golden Web. A compromised aura will only drain your energy and can manifest physical symptoms including infection, sudden illness, nausea, acute pain, headaches, and migraines. It could also lead to extreme mood swings and energy loss.

In a few days, your aura can recover through self-healing or a Reiki session. During the healing process, you will feel unwell, unconsciously desire for vital energy replenishment, and seek deep relaxation.

Most people are not aware of how to refill their universal life force energy source, so they just eat something for you to energize the body. Others may suck up the energy of others for you to feel recharged.

The thinning of your Golden Web can also lead to physical injuries felt in different parts of your body. If you don't seal these holes, it can affect your overall health in the long run. For example, leaking energy can lead to chronic fatigue if long-term cracks in a person's aura are not sealed off.

Furthermore, the leaks in your aura can increase your attachment to negative entities that may develop into more serious health problems later on. Attached entities steal your energy and introduce their negative markers to your energy field. As a result, you experience stronger psychological effects such as depression, fear, and anxiety.

If you haven't wondered where your negative emotions and thoughts are coming from, now is the best time to work on your leaking energy. Removing negative entities and energies from your energy field can help fix the holes and cracks in your aura. So, how do you repair your leaking energy?

How to Fix Energy Leaks

There are several methods to effectively fix the holes in your aura, but the most common is aura clearing. This method allows you to seal off the holes, tears, and cracks in your aura through your hands. Scan your aura using your hands at a 20-centimeter distance from your body. You can feel the breaks as holes, cold droughts, or pits.

If you think your hands are not sensitive enough to feel the breaks in your aura, you can use a crystal. Get your tower quartz crystal and hold it longitudinally from your head to your feet for you to clean your aura. Make sure the longitudinal passes are slowly applied to ensure it will work. Flick your quartz crystal over the bowl of salt water after every longitudinal pass to properly eliminate negative energies from your aura.

Repeat the process to cover your entire aura as there are several layers to cleanse. After the session, it's important to wash your crystal using another container of salt water to remove the negative energy. If not, you can clean your crystal by leaving it under direct sunlight for several hours to remove the dirty energy.

There are so many effective ways to clean and restore your aura. According to practitioners, the following methods can easily be done at home to fix your energy leaks. Just keep in mind the principles of balancing, protecting, energizing, healing, and cleansing the aura and other essential areas.

Before you start any method to clean and seal off your aura, make sure to ask for guidance from the Supreme Being so you can receive assistance, protection, and blessing. After the session, don't forget to give thanks to the divinity for helping you heal.

Now, for more tips to fix and restore your aura, you can do the rhythmic breathing and saltwater bath. The temperature of the water should be at least 40 degrees Celsius. Fill your hand with salt and pour it onto a container filled with water.

While you bathe in the salt water, say something like: "In God's name, I command all the unwanted energies of other beings to be removed from my body and aura. Redirect them into the earth for proper disposal."

after bathing in the salt water, you can recite this: "Divine Creator, I give thanks to You for restoring my aura, for filling it again with positive energy, for balancing my energetic fields, healing my body, and protecting me from all harm." Then practice rhythmic breathing for 10 cycles for you to recharge yourself.

If you want to cleanse and charge with nature, some of the activities you can do include the following:

- Swimming in the sea.

- Breathing in some fresh air.

- Basking in the sun.

- Walking under the rain.

Feel the natural force while doing any of these activities for you to cleanse and fix your aura. Let the negative energy flow out of your body while filling your chakras with positive energy so you can restore your aura.

You can also perform some visualizations such as the Golden Comb, the Whirlpool, hole patching, and more.

To visualize the Golden Comb, just imagine you're holding a comb with golden light. On your mind, imagine you are combing your aura using the golden light comb. Throw in all the negative energies into a violet flame then send it back to the ground.

If you want to try the Whirlpool, take a deep breath, and visualize yourself in a whirlpool filled with water-like energies from heaven. Then visualize the whirlpool picking up and carrying away all the negativity from your body to the universal ocean where it's dissolved without any trace.

The hole patching is done by mentally inspecting your aura and then locating the hole. Wash your aura with blue light for you to cleanse and close the hole. Visualize a thread and a needle with your preferred color to patch the hole. After fixing your aura, fill it with luminous golden light. Use your hands to gently smoothen the treated area.

It's truly amazing to simply use visual images to command the subconscious mind and heal the physical body. However, the results of these methods depend on your beliefs, imaginations, and skills in practicing energy healing.

Cleansing and restoring your aura should be done regularly to avoid long-lasting holes and cracks in your aura. It's as important as keeping your body clean and healthy. Paying attention to subtle fields can also help you achieve a higher psychological being.

If you understand that your subtle body doesn't only need physical healing but also spiritual healing, you will surely get the desired results after performing Reiki treatment. Your knowledge of fixing your leaking energy is an essential step in keeping your mind, body, and spirit in perfect balance.

Tips to Maintain a Clean and Closed Aura

Once you feel some weakness and reluctance in doing the activities that you usually do, it's time to check your physical body and its aura. Do not ignore the subtle signs of a leaking aura because it will only lead to serious medical conditions such as cancer and depression.

It's not enough to know how to close the holes in your aura, you also need to learn how to maintain it clean and smooth all the time. So, how do you keep your aura at its best condition? Here are some tips to maintain an aura that is free from negative energies and unwanted beings:

- Apply pressure on the affected area to expel the negative energies and restore your aura.

- Practice grounding and rooting daily or whenever it's needed.

- Learn and practice the micro cosmic orbit for you to help your energies flow and circulate better.

- Learn more about healing your chakras with crystals.

- Get some help from a Reiki healer who also use crystals to read auras.

Now if the lower chakras are completely open, your chakras might not be the problem but your energy flow that keeps them open. Some of the most common issues that keep the aura vulnerable are hedonistic tendencies, self-esteem problems, lack of discipline, and other serious personal issues that increase the flow of energy through your lower chakras.

It could also be another entity that is draining your energies. You can work with your practitioner for you to effectively get rid of these negative entities. Sometimes, you may also have multiple chords attached to a lot of people that also suck up on your energy. If that's the case, you can perform daily meditations for you to cut off negative people in your life.

Geshe Kelsang Gyatso's The Clear Light of Bliss indicates some helpful ideas on how to cure energy disorders and maintain a smooth aura in the long run. According to him, an ideal exercise to heal intense energy loss and restore the auric field is to practice meditation and visualize that your body is hollow or transparent.

Once you have made that visualization real, imagine your skin is full of small holes where the external environment joins the internal environment. In case of severe energy leaks, it's important to practice this meditation exercise daily for several weeks until you feel your aura has been restored.

To maintain healthy energy channels, build-up universal life force energy, and store Ki in the chakras, you can perform abdominal breathing, Qi Gong, embryonic breathing, and other similar exercises. The key is to fix your leaking energy before filling in your body with positive energy.

The potential danger of ignoring the problems in your aura is that it can lead to malfunctions in your root chakra and make you feel depressed, insane, or suicidal. This is why it's very important to recognize that energy is real and it may come and leave your body without your knowledge.

During stressful situations, Reiki treatment comes in handy. It can help you relax before you reach the level of burnouts and mental breakdowns. Every single day, you lose a significant amount of energy as you live your daily responsibilities in personal life and at work. You can't control the things around you, making it even more challenging to protect your energy from negative entities.

The integrity and strength in the layers of your auric field are essential in your overall energetic health. In fact, they serve as a foundation for your healing progress when treated with Reiki or other alternative medicine techniques.

Restoring your aura by closing leaks and cracks can bring back the integrity of your auric field while preventing your energy fields from becoming vulnerable to energy loss and negative energies. When restoring your aura, you have to be aware of your surroundings especially the nature of the auric field and energy you are fixing instead of distancing yourself from the flow of energy.

Although the hands are primarily used in correcting energy flows, unblocking chakras, clearing auric fields, closing energy leaks, and transferring universal life force energy, you are also using your entire being through your hands. Therefore, you need to be open and act like your whole self for you to address the issues in your energetic and auric fields.

Set aside the self-consciousness of your hands and other aspects of your materialistic self so you can focus on seeking clear channels to heal your body, mind, and spirit. Practice the techniques you've learned from this guide and view your aura as your whole being. This process is what you call transparency which is essential in understanding your healing needs.

Ultimately, the healing techniques should be performed with universal wisdom for you to achieve the healing outcome you exactly need. By cultivating this quality in practicing Reiki, you can learn more techniques that can address your problems in your auric field as well as your energy fields.

Signs You Have Negative Entities Attached to You

A negative energy or spirit attachment refers to a "clever" bodiless energy or spirit attached to the energy field or aura of a living person. Attachment entities are those that refuse to yield to death so they rather want to go on practicing certain behaviors in life. As a result, they continue to look for vulnerable human candidates whom they can "live" vicariously with.

The ultimate challenge in detecting spirit attachments is that they are hardly ever sensed. These sneaky entities are not physically felt nor seen, so you really have to work harder to identify if they have attached themselves to your body. Most people are not aware that there are negative spirits attached to them, making them even more vulnerable to energy problems.

The following are some tips to help you detect any negative energy or spirit attached to your body:

- Awareness. Perhaps, there's this weird feeling that makes you behave in an obsessive or unusual way. Your outlook may also turn somewhat hopeless while you feel depressed at the moment or for many years now.

Some of the mental and physical symptoms of spirit attachments include chronic tiredness, impulsive behavior, anger, inner voices saying negative things, addictions, poor memory, panic attacks, unexplained phobias, disturbing nightmares, and feeling another presence in certain places.

- Assessment. You need to undergo a direct assessment of your physical self and energy field for you to see if there are any negative entities or energies attached to your body. If you're suspecting there's a spirit attachment in your being, it's important to take decisive action.

- Detection. There are several effective methods to detect if there's something else living in your body. You can practice regression therapy, special meditations, examining dreams, muscle testing, using a pendulum, checking your aura in the mirror, automatic writing, journaling, and aura scanning.

However, the simplest method you can use is working with a Reiki practitioner to help you detect spirit attachments and removal.

- Identification. It's important to identify what is attached to you, whether it's simple negative energy or a sneaky negative entity or spirit. To do this, there are various self-tests you can try to see which one works for you. Ask your Reiki practitioner to guide you in identifying spirit attachments that are affecting your universal energy.

- Release. This is the final stage of identifying attachments of negative energies and entities in your body. It involves a cautious therapeutic release of spirit and energies attached to you. Some people are afraid to undergo this stage because they have been dealing with spirit attachments for many years, making it hard to let go.

Having negative energies in your body really sucks. It can put you in the worst mood while your body loses life force energy essential in boosting your immune system. Perhaps, you notice negative energies when you don't evoke the usual happiness you feel everyday.

Knowing that you're not yourself in the past few days is important in determining your physical, mental, emotional, and spiritual states. Once you get a hint that you're having some negative energies in your body, you can boost your mood through a Reiki session.

So, are you currently living in a complicated environment? If so, you are most likely to suffer from negative vibrations that diminish your well-being. You might also be living with people who are often sick, irritable, and tired. They can surely affect your overall health as well as how you perceive life.

It's important to live with people who know how to manage exhaustion and stress. There will surely be differences in your habits, but what's important is that you are able to handle them in a mature way. In addition, you should know when to sit down and talk about the issues you have at home. Good communication can help you settle your problems once and for all.

Another unhealthy habit that can put your chakras at risk is comparing yourself to others. Remember that each person has their own pace, it's not good to compare your achievements to other people. You might not be successful now, but you can always work harder to get the things you've always dreamed of.

How you treat yourself has a big impact on your spiritual self. When your spirit and mind are not balanced with your body, then your energy channels can go out of whack. It's important to focus on your goals, spend more time with your loved ones, work on your shortcomings, and stay committed to pursuing your passions.

Every time you feel low, shifting your perspectives and eliminating toxic elements and negative energies from your body can help you feel better and happier. When you enjoy life, it's easier to maintain your physical, mental, emotional, and spiritual health. At the same time, you can harmonize and balance your mind, body, and spirit while getting rid of the negative energy.

Conclusion

Reiki healing is one of the oldest forms of alternative medicine techniques that help clear negative influences from your body. It takes spiritual assistance from a Reiki healer for you to eliminate bad energies that keep people from living their life to the fullest.

This natural healing method can also help you build personal inner strength by making good decisions for yourself using spiritual practices instead of allowing negative influences such as drinking or overindulging. This guide will help you understand why you're feeling such emotions and easily falling sick despite exercising and eating a balanced diet.

Even if your body is getting enough nourishment, a compromised mental and emotional health can still make the physical body weak and vulnerable. Energetically bridging your energy through Reiki treatment is an essential step to heal your whole being.

This healing technique doesn't need physical touching to cure health issues. In fact, it can be done without closing physical proximity between the practitioner and the recipient. During a pandemic where people are required to practice social distancing, Reiki is one of the go-to healing therapies using distance Reiki sessions.

As long as you're comfortable and at ease, Reiki can provide you with healing benefits, unlike other alternative medicine techniques. However, it's important to develop a deep connection with your practitioner for you to achieve a higher level of spiritual experience need to restore harmony and balance in your mind, body, and spirit.

Once the foundation has been established, it's easier for the practitioner to work on the healing process. During the session, you may visualize a thunderstorm followed by a clear blue sky. Also, you will feel deeply understood and cared for by someone. Your senses are suddenly animated and you feel like everything around you is clear and sensible.

You might be scared to try Reiki for the first time, this is why you are given this guide to overcome your fears as a beginner in energy healing. The endless energy flowing through your body, mind, and spirit is a great subject to study. With proper education about natural healing and its potential benefits to your whole being, it's easier to know whether this technique will work on you or not.

If you're feeling down lately, it's best to talk to a Reiki healer to help you determine what is causing the sudden low mood. However, if you're curious enough how to perform this healing technique on your own, you can simply follow the instructions provided in the previous chapters about how to perform self-Reiki.

You will be surprised by how the quality of your life quickly changes after doing a self-healing session. Don't forget to practice meditation regularly for you to clam your mind, relax your body, and soother your soul. So, are you ready to explore the infinite benefits of Reiki healing? Start practicing it today to see the huge difference it can make in your life.